A Primer on
Systemic Lupus Erythematosus

Amita Aggarwal MD DM
Professor and Head
Department of Clinical Immunology and Rheumatology
Sanjay Gandhi Postgraduate Institute of Medical Sciences
Lucknow, India

Anisur Rahman MD PhD
Professor of Rheumatology
Division of Medicine
Faculty of Medical Sciences
University College, London, UK

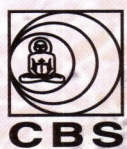

CBS

CBS Publishers & Distributors Pvt Ltd

New Delhi • Bengaluru • Chennai • Kochi • Kolkata • Mumbai
Hyderabad • Jharkhand • Nagpur • Patna • Pune • Uttarakhand

A Primer on
Systemic Lupus Erythematosus

ISBN: 978-93-90046-04-1

Copyright © Indian Rheumatology Assosication

First Edition: 2021

Published by Satish Kumar Jain and produced by Varun Jain for

CBS Publishers & Distributors Pvt Ltd

4819/XI Prahlad Street, 24 Ansari Road, Daryaganj, New Delhi 110 002, India.
Ph: 23289259, 23266861, 23266867 Website: www.cbspd.com
Fax: 011-23263014   e-mail: delhi@cbspd.com; cbspubs@airtelmail.in.

Corporate Office: 204 FIE, Industrial Area, Patparganj, Delhi 110 092

Ph: 4934 4934   Fax: 4934 4935   e-mail: publishing@cbspd.com; publicity@cbspd.com

Branches

- **Bengaluru:** Seema House 2975, 17th Cross, K.R. Road, Banasankari 2nd Stage, Bengaluru 560 070, Karnataka
  Ph: +91-80-26771678/79   Fax: +91-80-26771680   e-mail: bangalore@cbspd.com
- **Chennai:** 7, Subbaraya Street, Shenoy Nagar, Chennai 600 030, Tamil Nadu
  Ph: +91-44-26680620, 26681266   Fax: +91-44-42032115   e-mail: chennai@cbspd.com
- **Kochi:** 42/1325, 1326, Power House Road, Opp KSEB, Kochi 682 018, Kerala, India
  Ph: +91-484-4059061-65,67   Fax: +91-484-4059065   e-mail: kochi@cbspd.com
- **Kolkata:** 6/B, Ground Floor, Rameswar Shaw Road, Kolkata-700014 (West Bengal), India
  Ph: +91-33-2289-1126, 2289-1127, 2289-1128   e-mail: kolkata@cbspd.com
- **Mumbai:** 83-C, Dr E Moses Road, Worli, Mumbai-400018, Maharashtra
  Ph: +91-22-24902340/41   Fax: +91-22-24902342   e-mail: mumbai@cbspd.com

Representatives

- Hyderabad   0-9885175004
- Patna   0-9334159340
- Jharkhand   0-9811541605
- Pune   0-9623451994
- Nagpur   0-9421945513
- Uttarakhand 0-9716462459

Printed at Magic International Pvt. Ltd., Greater Noida, UP, India

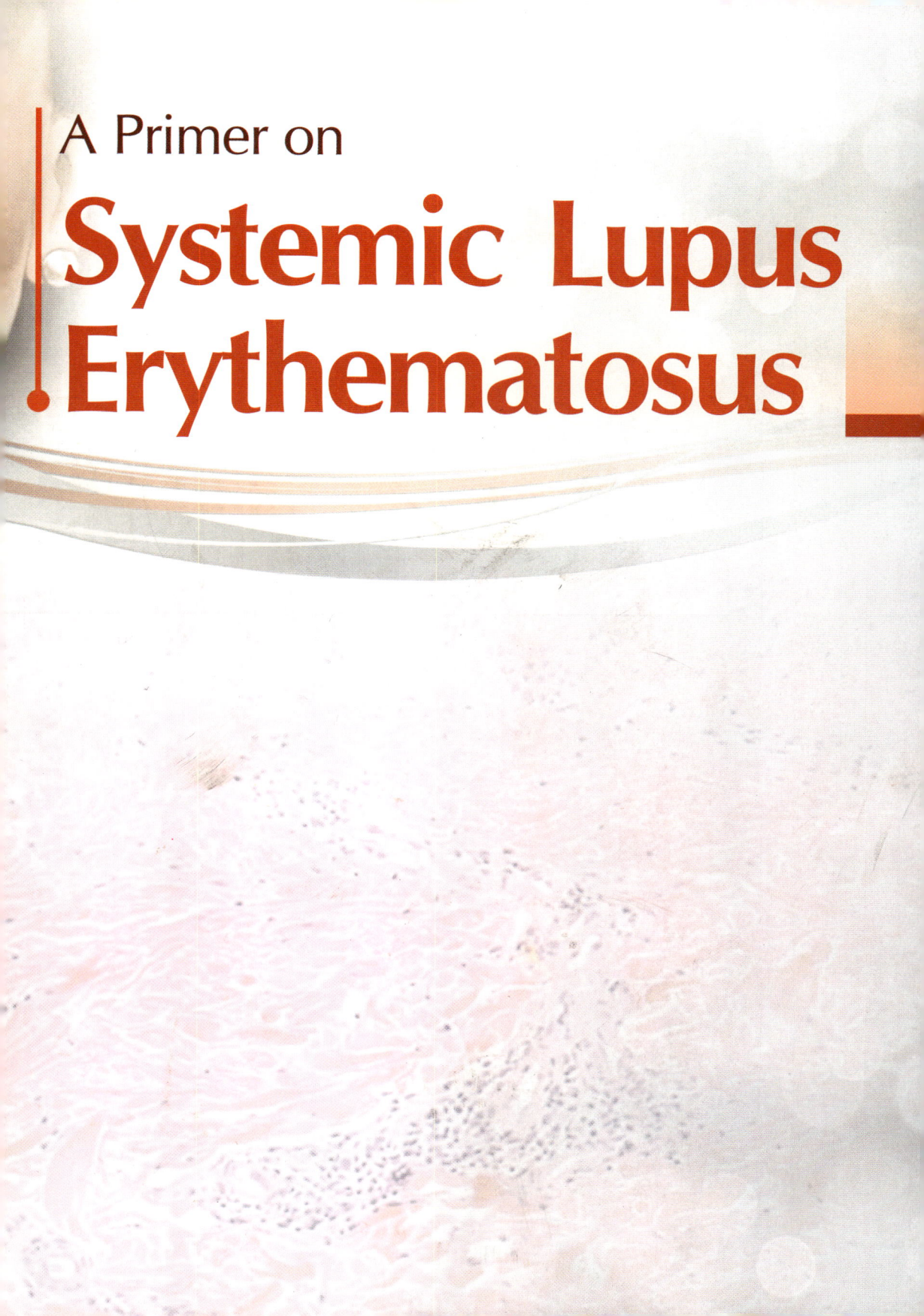

A Primer on

Systemic Lupus Erythematosus

Preface

When we were approached to edit a book on systemic lupus erythematosus (SLE) by Indian Rheumatology Association, we very gladly agreed. There were several reasons for it. First, 'lupus' is one of the most fascinating and challenging diseases in the field of rheumatology. Second, knowledge about this disease in India and in several countries in the region is relatively limited. Third, the clinicians who deal with this disease face a wide variety of challenges and are in great need of guidance from peers.

Lupus is truly a multisystem disease, so that patients can present with myriad clinical features affecting different organs or tissues either simultaneously or sequentially. Thus, patients with this disease present to not only to any subspecialist in medicine, but also to practitioners of other specialties, such as dermatologists, obstetricians, etc. It has rightly been said that if one knows lupus, one knows the whole of medicine. The presentation can also vary from a mild niggle in the form of a minor skin rash to pronounced hair loss to a catastrophic, life-threatening illness, such as rapidly progressive renal failure or a stroke. It can simulate a wide variety of other illnesses, leading to missed diagnosis. Thus, the correct diagnosis, i.e. of systemic lupus erythematosus, is often made only when a smart physician decides to think beyond the ordinary, e.g. deciding to look for a link between the current manifestations in one organ system with a past illness in another organ system. Once one starts to connect the dots, often the diagnosis is easily apparent—making one feel a bit foolish for not having thought of it earlier.

However, the story does not end with the diagnosis. It is not unusual for the treating doctor—whether a clinical immunologist, rheumatologist or an organ specialist—to face several therapeutic dilemmas. Should I treat the minor involvement with steroids or not? Are immunosuppressive drugs needed or not? Are biologicals needed? Add to that the dilemmas related to short- and long-term prognosis, patients' questions about pregnancy and occupation—and we have a full conundrum.

Lupus is enigmatic not only for clinicians, but also for biologists. Being a prototype autoimmune disease, lupus is one of the most widely studied model for the study of autoimmunity. Whereas autoantibodies present in the circulation and in inflamed tissues represent the final agents of pathogenesis, almost every facet of the immune system may be dysfunctional in SLE. Thus, B cells, T cells, monocytes, complement and cytokines have all been studied in humans with lupus and in animal models of the disease. All of these immune components are potential targets for new biologic agents.

This book begins with an article by Prof Anand N Malaviya—one of the first persons to work on lupus in India. This piece is a rendition of his journey over nearly four decades beginning with the first recognition of patients with lupus in India, and of the trials and tribulations of managing patients with lupus. This is followed by articles on various manifestations of lupus and its treatment. These have been written with a clinical perspective, addressing the dilemmas faced in managing patients with lupus. Many articles include case vignettes to add a real-life feel. Issues such as balancing the pros and cons of therapy and how to improve long-term outcome have also been discussed. The issue ends with a patient's perspective of the disease.

We are grateful to our contributors, all of whom are active workers in the field, who very kindly agreed to take time out of their busy schedules to write for this book. Our sincere thanks are all also due to Dr Rudrarpan Chatterjee, who helped us with proofreading. We do hope that the readers of this book **A Primer on Systemic Lupus Erythematosus** will find our effort worthwhile.

Amita Aggarwal
Anisur Rahman

Contributors List

Abdulrahman Alrashid MD
Clinical Research Fellow
Louise Coote Lupus Unit
Guy's Hospital
London, UK

Abhishek Zanwar MD DM
Consultant Rheumatologist
Ruby Hall Clinic
Pune, India

Amita Aggarwal MD DM
Professor and Head
Department of Clinical Immunology and
Rheumatology
Sanjay Gandhi Postgradaute Institute of
Medical Sciences
Lucknow, India
aa.amita@gmail.com

Anand N Malaviya MD FRCP
Former Head, Department of Medicine
Chief of Clinical Immunology and
Rheumatology Services
All India Institute of Medical Sciences
New Delhi, India

Head, Department of Rheumatology
ISIC Superspeciality Hospital
Vasant Kunj, New Delhi, India
anand_malaviya@yahoo.com

Anisur Rahman MD PhD
Professor
Department of Rheumatology
Division of Medicine, Faculty of Medical
Sciences, University college, London UK
anisur.rahman@ucl.ac.uk

Avinash Jain MD DM
Assistant Professor (Rheumatology)
Department of Medicine
Sawai Mansingh Medical College and Hospital
Jaipur, India

Benzeeta Pinto MD DM
Department of Clinical Immunology and
Rheumatology
St. John's National Academy of Health Sciences
Bengaluru, India

Bidyut Kumar Das MD FRCP
Professor and Head
Department of Rheumatology
SCB Medical College, Cuttack, India
bidyutdas@hotmail.com

Bushra Khan
bushrakhan20@gmail.com

Chengappa Kavadichanda G MD DM
Assistant Professor
Department of Clinical Immunology
JIPMER, Puducherry, India

David P D'Cruz MD FRCP
Consultant Rheumatologist
Louise Coote Lupus Unit
Guy's Hospital
London
david.d'cruz@kcl.ac.uk

Jyoti Bakshi MD
Department of Rheumatology
Division of Medicine, Faculty of Medical
Sciences, University college, London UK

Keerthi Talari Bommakanti MD DM
Consultant Rheumatologist
Yashoda Hospitals, Secunderabad
Telangana, India

Latika Gupta MD DM
Assistant Professor
Department of Clinical Immunology and
Rheumatology
Sanjay Gandhi Postgraduate Institute of
Medical Sciences
Lucknow, India

Liza Rajasekhar MD
Professor and Head
Department of Clinical Immunology and
Rheumatology
Nizam's Institute of Medical Sciences
Hyderabad, Telangana, India
lizarajasekhar@gmail.com

Naman Jain MD
Registrar
Department of Rheumatology
Manipal Hospital, Bengaluru, India

Ramnath Misra MD FRCP
Professor and Head
Department of Rheumatology
Kalinga Institute of Medical Sciences
Bhubaneshwar, India
rnmisra2000@gmail.com

Rudrarpan Chatterjee MD
Senior Resident
Department of Clinical Immunology and
Rheumatology
Sanjay Gandhi Postgraduate Institute of
Medical Sciences
Lucknow, India

Sanat Phatak MD DM
Associate Consultant (Rheumatology)
Department of Medicine and Diabetes Unit
KEM Hospital Research Centre
Pune, India

Saumya Ranjan Tripathy MD DM
Assistant Professor
Department of Rheumatology
SCB Medical College
Cuttack, India

Sujata Sawhney MD MRCP CCST (UK)
Senior Consultant, Pediatric and
Adolescent Rheumatology
Division of Pediatric Rheumatology
Institute of Child Health
Sir Ganga Ram Hospital, New Delhi, India
drsujatasawhney@gmail.com

Yogesh Mann Singh MD DM
Consultant and Head
Department of Rheumatology
Manipal Hospital, Old airport road
Bengaluru, India
yogeshmann@gmail.com

Vineeta Shobha MD DM
Professor and Head
Department of Clinical Immunology and
Rheumatology
St. John's National Academy of Health Sciences
Bengaluru, India
vineeta.s@stjohns.in

Vir Singh Negi MD DM
Professor and Head
Department of Clinical Immunology
JIPMER, Puducherry, India
vsnegi22@yahoo.co.in

Contents

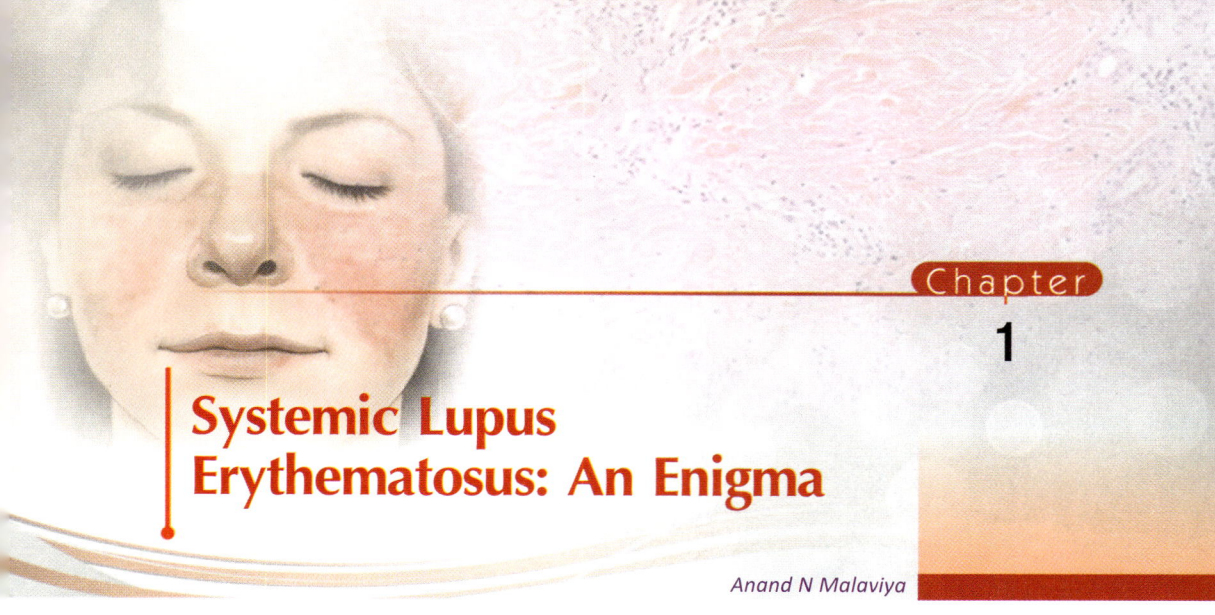

Systemic Lupus Erythematosus: An Enigma

Anand N Malaviya

INTRODUCTION

I am honoured on being invited to write the opening article a monograph on systemic lupus erythematosus (SLE). For setting the agenda for the topic under discussion, I shall like to take the present day practicing rheumatologists back in time, to the India of yester-years, more precisely the year 1968. That was a socially, politically, commercially, scientifi-cally and academically a different India. That was a 'socialist' India with a 'closed' economy where there was a complete ban on imports of any item from the smallest (e.g. sewing needles) to the largest (e.g. cars). The 'License Raj' ruled the roost. There were mostly single or at the most a few manufacturers for items like motorbike, scooters and cars. Locally manufactured medical instruments for even a basic-level clinical laboratory were woefully below standard. To buy even a small item like a good microscope, would entail at least 50 clearances from different government offices. Bribery was at every step for obtaining the licence. This was the scenario when I returned from Boston, fully trained in the clinical and laboratory aspects of what we know today as systemic immunoinflammatory rheumatic diseases (SIRD).

This group of diseases were labelled 'the collagen diseases' or 'connective tissue diseases' in those days. I had applied for a faculty position at the All India Institute of Medical Sciences (AIIMS), New Delhi from Boston, USA. When I reached Delhi (September 1968) I met the then AIIMS Director, a legendary physician Prof Kushwant Lal Wig. A small digression—in those days there were no quotas, only merit was the consideration! I had only 2 publications but they were in the 2 highest-rated journals of the time ('The Lancet' and 'Journal of Experimental Medicine'). That was considered sufficient for appointment to the Faculty of AIIMS without interview! My first meeting with the then AIIMS Director, is worth mentioning in the context of SLE. He asked me about my academic interest and how do I plan to develop the field of my clinical and research interest ('collagen diseases'). Then, he thoughtfully added "You know these diseases are not common in India; in my career I have seen only a few patients where I could make a clinical diagnosis of SLE".[1] Then, he advised me to meet Prof V Ramalingaswamy (head of the department of pathology, possibly one of the greatest medical researchers and scientists produced by our country). "Because he is the laboratory man and will help you. As there will be very few patients with 'collagen diseases', you can utilise your time in setting up a good autoimmune laboratory". I came out of the Director's office on 'Cloud Nine'! No interview, no nothing, became Assistant Professor in 10 minutes. Those were the AIIMS days; difficult to believe!

INTERNATIONAL VISITORS

In New England Medical Centre, Boston, performing anti-nuclear antibody test was damn easy. Linda (the laboratory technician) was always ready to help. Mouse liver sections on slides were ready, fluorescein conjugates were on the shelf courtesy Sigma Lab, Detroit, state-of-the-art fluorescent microscope was at hand. I truly believed that performing IFT-ANA would be the easiest test to set-up in India. I was wrong. How to get mouse liver? How to make frozen sections, where is the freezing microtome and who will cut the sections? Where is the fluorescein conjugate? Imports of any reagents in India were banned or needed special permit—those were the days of socialistic India, nothing was available. Again, God (and Prof Ramalingaswamy) smiled on me! A few months after I joined AIIMS, two famous clinical immunologists from Melbourne, Australia Senga Whittingham and Ian Mackay[2] visited AIIMS. They took upon themselves to help explain all the small gadgets and items that I needed in the laboratory and got them fabricated from the AIIMS workshop (Figs 1.1a to d), made me use the AIIMS animal house to produce anti-gamma globulin

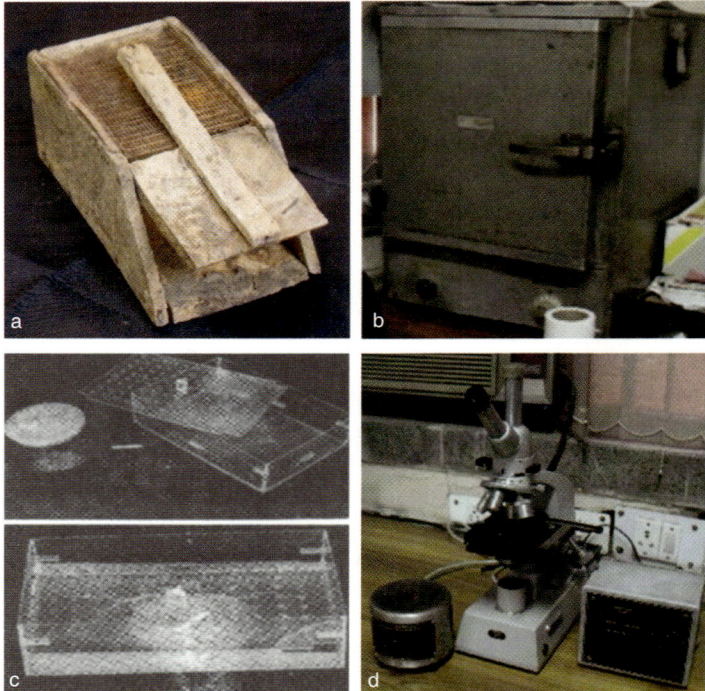

Figs 1.1a to d: Instruments in the clinical immunology laboratory of AIIMS, New Delhi, 1972. (a) Locally available mouse trap for rodent liver section to be used for ANA test; (b) A locally made laboratory incubator; (c) Plexiglass-ANA slide washer with false bottom and a magnetic stirrer; (d) A monocular epifluorescence microscope for reading IFT-ANA

antibodies, promised me to send some fluorescein dye through the next visitor from Australia. The famous British Clinical Immunologist EJ Holborow (Editor of a famous book of those days 'Standardization in Immunofluorescence' January 1, 1970), had earlier taught me (in an autoimmune workshop held in Lausanne, Switzerland) how to make the fluorescein conjugates and conduct the indirect fluorescent test for the antinuclear antibodies (IFT-ANA). I was all set! In 1975, another famous clinical immunologist and an expert in the *Crithidia luciliae*-based indirect immunofluorescence test for the detection of antibody against double-stranded-DNA (dsDNA), TE Feltkamp (from The Netherlands)[3] visited AIIMS and brought *Crithidia luciliae* in a test-tube culture nicely incubated in his inner coat pocket! Prof Ramesh Kumar, Department of Microbiology, AIIMS and a very dear friend and collaborator, successfully grew and set up the *Crithidia luciliae* culture line that we used for several decades. The fourth visitor who was instrumental in furthering the working of the AIIMS clinical immunology laboratory was Stratis Avrameas, a French Immunologist [the discoverer of the enzyme-linked immunoassay (ELISA) technique].[4] He brought a pack of polysterine plates with small wells (called 'ELISA plates') and sat down in the clinical immunology laboratory of AIIMS and demonstrated the ELISA technique step-by-step, to a brilliant youngster working in my laboratory Ram Nath Misra. The addition of the ELISA test by Avrameas-Misra made AIIMS clinical immunology laboratory a top laboratory in India for investigating 'connective tissue diseases' (the name that we used for several years to come).

THE IMMUNOLOGY CLINIC

'What is there in a name' is an oft-repeated cliché! In the context of 'collagen diseases' actually it meant a lot. Armed with a decent laboratory for autoantibodies, in early 1970s it was imperative to start a clinic exclusively for the diagnosis, treatment and follow-up of patients with these diseases. Should it be named 'autoimmune diseases' clinic; 'arthritis clinic'; 'rheumatology clinic'? Objections were made by the department of dermatology and orthopaedics; it was their domain! Prof Ramalingaswamy suggested calling it 'Immunology clinic' (with a back-up of the 'clinical immunology' laboratory). Thus, the clinic was started in 1973. (In retrospect, the best name could have been 'connective tissue diseases clinic', but that was destiny). It was simply amazing (Figs 1.2 and 1.3); within a few months we saw a number of cases where we could make the diagnosis of SLE along with a smattering of a few patients with dermatomyositis (rash resembling SLE). With the laboratory backup, within a few years we published several large series of patients with these diseases.[5–10] But, being fascinated with lupus our group published some of the largest series on this disease from India.[6,11–13] In 1983, during one of the DRA meetings, Prof Wig also came to attend (he was a patron in those days). To his greatness, he told me 'you have done a good job, you have shown that lupus is not uncommon in India, as I used to believe'!

Patients are the Best Teachers

The Triumphs and Travails of Treating Lupus

In the beginning lupus was easy to recognise and diagnose. Young woman with photosensitive facial rash (not crossing the nasolabial fold), hair loss, off and on fever, arthritis/arthralgia, mouth ulcers with a positive ANA, was SLE. We would prescribe prednisolone and chloroquine (in those days hydroxychloroquine was not available in India) and soon

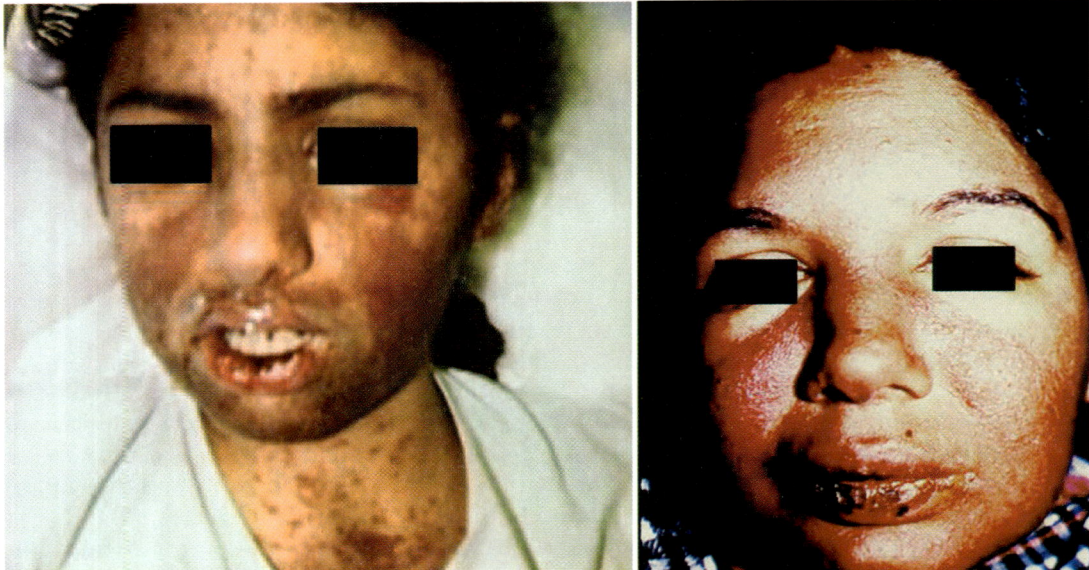

Figs 1.2 and 1.3: Patients of SLE from early days in AIIMS

the patient would be better on low-dose (5 to 7.5 mg) prednisolone. All appeared hunky-dory!

Then, (Late) Prof Manmohan Singh Ahuja, the then Head of the Department of Medicine, at AIIMS, requested me to see the daughter of his friend, a Professor of English at the Delhi University. A nice young woman of 21 years of age with ~2 months of typical features of SLE–photosensitive facial rash, off and on fever, a few mouth ulcers, joint pains but one noticeable unusual feature that I could only understand in retrospect was, the extremely talkative nature often suddenly lapsing in out-of-context questions. It was only after several years that I understood what my teachers used to call 'young crazy girls with headaches' as one of the presenting features of lupus. Our home-made IFT-ANA test was positive in high titre (by that time my laboratory had not started the home-made *Crithidia*-IFT testing and anti-sera to C3, C4 was just being raised in the goats in the Animal House of the AIIMS). With the diagnosis of SLE and patient education about avoiding sun (and UV light) exposure, cold exposure and regular exercise, she was prescribed chloroquine and low-dose prednisolone with immediate and dramatic improvement. But, her talkative nature was unchanged. I do not remember exactly but somewhere between 3 and 4 months down-the-lane, her mother called me that she is all 'swollen up from head to toe' with breathlessness! The mother told me that as she was feeling absolutely fine, she joined her friends for a holiday trip to the hill station, Naini Taal frolicking around in open sun for several days! Urgent admission and workup revealed '4+' proteinuria, hypertension and breathlessness. There were no nephrologists in AIIMS at that time and renal biopsy was out-of-the question in early 1970s. I took courage and gave what I had learnt in Boston—'pulse steroid' (dexamethasone to be precise) with 'pulse' cyclophosphamide. With the moral support of the HOD, I went ahead with this treatment. It is interesting to recall that methylprednisolone was not available in India at that time. Instead, we used to give dexamethasone 'pulse'.

Along with the supportive measures including diuretics, she responded quickly and the patient and family were grateful. Lo-and-behold, a few weeks down the lane, she was readmitted with high fever, altered sensorium and deteriorating vital signs. Investigations showed extensive bilateral pneumonia, she succumbed. But for the support of Prof Ahuja, the HOD, I would have been summarily dismissed from the AIIMS faculty. 'How can any doctor use cancer drugs for a benign disease like lupus', colleagues were asking! Big lesson learnt—counselling of the patients and the family members regarding lifestyle changes for lupus patients should be an integral part of the management. Secondly, the drugs we often use in desperation are nasty substances, be very careful.

Then is the fascinating story of a patient of mine since 1980 (starting from AIIMS, New Delhi), who is now more like a family friend. I consider her to be my 'teacher' whom I have admired the most. She has taught me more about lupus than any other teacher or textbook. She, an attractive 22-year-old airhostess, presented with the onset of joint pains of a few weeks' duration, soon followed by what she called 'muscle failure' (on examination severe proximal muscle weakness, wheel-chair bound) that had progressed rapidly, along with a photosensitive facial rash and history of Raynaud's phenomenon. There was past history of thrombocytopenic purpura (diagnosed as ITP–1978, treated with prednisolone with complete recovery). Muscle enzymes and a biopsy from the quadriceps confirmed 'inflammatory myositis'. Facial rash, Raynaud's and strongly positive anti-nuclear antibody—all pointed out to the diagnosis of an 'overlap connective tissue disease' with prominent features of inflammatory muscle disease and lupus. Having published the first paper ever on the use of low-dose methotrexate in an inflammatory rheumatic disease (in those days the name was collagen disease),[14] I considered myself an 'expert' in this disease. I was excited to treat her with my newly discovered indication of methotrexate for this disease, combined with prednisolone.

There was some anxiety about 'another cancer drug' in a 'benign disease' but with the full backing of the HOD, the treatment was initiated with prompt response and an appreciative patient. All was well till a few months later she was admitted with acute breathlessness. Fortunately, she recovered from severe bacterial pneumonia and was back to almost normal health in a few months. To cut the long clinical story of decades short, she has successfully battled renal involvement with facial swelling (1985) treated with glucocorticoids (GC) and azathioprine, recurrent lose motions with occasional severe diarrhea (she calls it 'weak belly') with symptomatic treatments, transient depression (problems in personal life-related to disease in the year 1992), recurrent disease flares controlled with low-dose methotrexate and occasional jacking-up of GC; long-term adverse effects of GC treatment including hypertension (still on treatment), cataract (operated—in the year 1998), multifocal osteonecrosis (requiring bilateral hip replacement years 1998, and 2000), small bones in the feet osteonecrosis causing advanced foot deformities 1998 onwards (requiring special footwear) with difficulty in walking, osteoporosis (despite treatment) with increasing kyphoscoliosis from the year 2000 onwards (severe pains in the whole of the back, neck, upper chest, difficulty to dress herself properly). She also developed carcinoma cervix in 2006 (pan-hysterectomy operation with radiation) leading to lymphatic blockage and severe lower limb oedema treated with physical means, episode of myocardial infarction in 2009 (triple vessel disease) that required stenting, recurrence of carcinoma cervix (2012) again treated with radiation with worsening of the leg oedema and difficulty in footwear and walking. Knees are waiting to be replaced, one episode of scary 'red urine'

5 years ago, that turned out to be beeturia (had eaten beet-root salad in the dinner the night before)! The latest problem was in early 2018 when she called 'I am unable to stand or walk'! Was it the recurrence of myositis? Detailed workup excluded any inflammatory muscle disease. A colleague with interest in SLE suggested to treat her empirically with intravenous immunoglobulin (for any occult lupus activity, any muscle inflammation that could not be picked up by the usual investigations) and denosumab for the severe osteoporosis that she has been having (treated with teriparatide in the past). The effect of this treatment was magical; she stood up and started walking within 2 weeks. She is back to her managerial work full time. Just to summarize, the drugs that she has taken over the years at variable doses included hydroxychloroquine, GC, methotrexate, azathioprine, calcium supplementations, bisphosphonates, teriparatide and denosumab, anti-hypertensives, ACE-inhibitors, low-dose aspirin, vitamin D_3, folic acid and other supportive measures. Socially, she has been single after a few years of marriage. She did not try for pregnancy due to her illness. Present status: In her mid-fifties, she is fully employed, still manages herself in a house where she lives alone. The lesson, in lupus is 'never give-up'; it is a question of the life of human being. Soon after the submission of this manuscript for publication, she developed resistant heart failure due to ischemic cardiomyoapthy and succumbed to the illness.

Another patient was a real VIP, daughter of a top Bureaucrat in Government of India. The year was 1987. Our Director (AIIMS) asked me to take care of the patient who was diagnosed 'A collagen disease' by a senior physician in the central government health service. The diagnosis appeared correct; she had all the typical features of SLE of mild superficial, mucocutaneous, arthritis variety of the disease. By then, besides IFT-ANA, my laboratory had started the home-made *Crithidia*-anti-dsDNA antibody IFT as well as C3 and C4 levels. All these tests confirmed SLE. The response to chloroquine (hydroxychloroquine was still not available) and prednisolone was dramatic. Director, my HOD as well as the patient and her family highly appreciated our efforts. The only problem was that one of her close relatives, a medical doctor, conveyed to the family members that the treating doctor at AIIMS (i.e. me) is a 'mouse doctor', only does experiments and he may be using your daughter as a guinea pig! Hats-off to her father, he was steadfast and shunned her away; to say the least, the patient did well over the next several years.

In 1996, when I was abroad, she developed clinical features of meningitis (high fever, severe headaches, vomiting). Unfortunately, instead of immediately going to AIIMS, she went to her doctor-relative mentioned above. The only news that I got later-on was that she was given cyclophosphamide by her doctor-relative. Soon after this 'treatment' the patient died! The question still lingers in my mind whether she had septic meningitis that was neither diagnosed nor treated. I learnt another lesson—patients must be properly counselled about what speciality of physicians they should approach for advice. Lupus has many faces— 'multi-headed hydra'—only a trained clinical immunologist–rheumatologist would be able to recognise the different presentations, different subcategories and protean complications of lupus in different organ systems.

EARLY PUBLICATIONS IN THE FIELD OF SLE FROM INDIA

By 1990s, 'Immunology Clinic' at AIIMS, New Delhi had one of the largest number of SLE patients under follow-up, in the country. In this regard, a comment by Sir Ravinder Maini (the first user of a monoclonal antibody—infliximab—in clinical medicine in rheumatoid arthritis to be precise) during his visit to AIIMS in the 1980s was interesting; "I have never seen so many SLE patients in a single clinic on the same day"! He encouraged us to publish SLE data. His advice was taken seriously. Over the next several years 51 research papers were published from the 'Clinical Immunology' Division of the Department of Medicine at the AIIMS, New Delhi, some of them are being cited.[15-23] One notable paper was on the prevalence of SLE in the population.[13] The survey was based upon the screening of the population for anti-nuclear antibody; those found positive were then clinically evaluated. In 91,888 persons surveyed, there were three cases of SLE, giving a point prevalence of 3.2 per 100,000 (95% CI = 0–6.86 per 100,000). The reported prevalence of SLE ranged from 14 to 60 per 100,000. Thus, the prevalence of SLE in India was comparatively low. Another key paper was on the survival of patients with SLE in India,[24] that showed significant reduction of lifespan in SLE patients. The problem of shortened life expectancy, despite many advances in the treatment of SLE, remains a major unmet need till date.[25]

THAT UNCOMFORTABLE/INSECURE FEELING ABOUT LUPUS

With 5 decades of having evaluated, diagnosed and managed SLE patients, I still feel apprehensive when I see a patient with this disease. It is one of the most complicated and confusing diseases with a broad spectrum of presentations and disease courses. The worst part is that there are hardly any 'markers of prognosis' and nothing to forecast the future course of the disease in a given patient. Will she remain mild, superficial, mucocutaneous, musculoskeletal lupus? Will she develop renal lupus, neuropsychiatric or severe neurological lupus or acute toxic SLE? What haematological manifestations will be the most troublesome in her disease course? The skin lesions are that of SLE or some unrelated problem? The pleural or pericardial effusion (or both) is tuberculous or, part of lupus serositis? The fluctuating liver enzymes indicate lupoid hepatitis or are these due to the prescribed drugs? The recurrent abdominal pains and bloating in a young woman are due to Koch's abdomen or mesenteric vasculitis due to lupus? Seizure is related to the anti-phospholipid syndrome or lupus brain involvement? Several symptoms of lupus (fever, weight loss) as well as symptoms of organ involvement (especially lung, neurological, gastrointestinal symptoms, others), may also be seen in infections.

It is one of the most difficult clinical exercises to differentiate 'SLE involvement' from 'infection'. Yet, this distinction is vital for appropriate treatment. Pains in different joints (including the localised pains in the carpal or the tarsal joints) are due to synovitis flare or due to ischemic necrosis of the bone? The treatment of these two manifestations is so different that it becomes imperative to have an exact diagnosis. Thanks to the newer imaging techniques, it has become easier to get the correct diagnosis. A generally accepted feature of SLE is that after the initial 2 years the 'disease breeds true' for the rest of the life. It means that the disease may show changing manifestations and organ involvement pattern early in its course. Then, after 2 years the disease pattern remains more-or-less the same. So, a mild superficial mucocutaneous, arthritis lupus may remain with the same pattern with some fluctuation in the disease course. A polyserositic lupus may remain with the same pattern with fluctuations. Predominantly haematological SLE would remain in that category for most of its course. Lupus nephritis or a CNS lupus would mostly follow the same pattern and a lupus with 'difficult pregnancy-related issues' will likely to have the same problem with every pregnancy. But, this adage is not sacrosanct; the treating rheumatologist, neurologist, nephrologist, gastroenterologist, ophthalmologist may be in for a surprise—a stable patient for years may suddenly develop an entirely new manifestations without any reason or warnings! That also brings in a basic rule related to the management of SLE. With protean manifestations, it is mandatory for the patients to be best treated by a team of specialists. However, it is imperative that the management team leader must be a rheumatologist.

Where are the drugs for treating SLE? But, All is not that Gloomy!

It is rather amazing that till date, there are only 2 FDA (USA) approved specific drugs for the treatment of lupus namely; glucocorticoids and belimumab. And, the pity is that the latter is not available in India! All the other drugs being used in SLE are 'off-label', mostly borrowed from the other 'sister' rheumatic diseases. Trials after trials with newer and mechanistically promising drugs, have failed to meet the primary end-points. However, in routine rheumatology practice the treatment of lupus is fairly standardised and most patients are quite well managed. Certain basic rules related to lifestyle along with what we would like to call 'basic background treatment' are good enough for most SLE patients with no major issues. A good healthy lifestyle is essential for their management. They must be repeatedly counselled about protection from Sun (ultraviolet) light (clothing, sun-screen lotions and avoiding outdoor lifestyle; avoiding hill-stations where ultra-violet exposure is very high). They must be strongly advised about balanced diet and maintaining weight, regular workouts with impact exercises (to prevent osteoporosis), staying away from smoking, and stringently preventing cold exposures (Raynaud's phenomenon is a problem for most of them). Every patient with SLE must be prescribed the 'basic background treatment'. It consists of hydroxychloroquine (HCQ),[26] adequate dose of vitamin D_3,[27] folic acid supplementation, especially if they are taking methotrexate[28] and vitamin B_{12} supplementation (specific for Indians who are primarily vegetarian),[29] and natural (not supplementary) calcium in the form of calcium-rich diet (list easily available at 'Google' on-line). Low-dose aspirin is also recommended in most patients[30,31] because several autopsy reports show widespread microthromboses in different organs of lupus patients of long-standing especially if associated with anti-phospholipid syndrome.[32] Joint and muscle symptoms are common and require non-steroidal anti-inflammatory drugs (NSAIDs) with caution as rarely aseptic meningitis is reported with their use.[33] For reasons that are still not fully understood, celecoxib seems to be more effective and beneficial in SLE than other NSAIDs.[34]

The positive effect of statins in systemic autoimmune rheumatic diseases including SLE seems well accepted,[35] especially because of increased cardiovascular risk in such diseases including SLE.[36] Over the years, slowly but surely, the benefits of low-dose methotrexate (LD-MTX) in controlling several SLE manifestations have been recognised including its high efficacy in inflammatory arthritis in SLE, skin lesions and serositis.[37,38] This had led to the waning popularity of azathioprine. But, in recent times the drug that has really changed the outcome of lupus patients is mycophenolate mofetil (MMF). It seems to be effective in controlling most of the manifestations of SLE. In my decades of experience with SLE, I feel that MMF has had the biggest therapeutic impact on the treatment of SLE after HCQ. The other major therapeutic change that has drastically improved the lupus treatment is the improved understanding of how to use glucocorticoids (GC) in this disease. In olden days, as a rule, every patient, irrespective of the type of SLE, was prescribed GC as a 'knee-jerk' reaction! Thanks to Michelle Petri, an SLE specialist at the Johns Hopkins Medical School,

Baltimore, USA, GC use in SLE is now shunned completely except in severe/desperate situations. Even in such situations, Petri has propounded a simple rule—'hit-hard and run-away'! A recent paper provides the proof.[39] Over the years she has proved that this approach for the use of GC in SLE saves life; prevents the horrible GC-related long-term complications e.g. multifocal-osteonecrosis and generalized atherosclerosis-related complications. This simple treatment philosophy has brought about dramatic change in the outcome of SLE patients. But, belimumab is still not available in India. Colleagues working abroad tell us that this drug is another 'game changer' for the patients with mild to moderate form of SLE who are not well controlled with the drugs mentioned above. Though ritiximab did not show benefit in trials, it is widely used in difficult situations and has shown 70–80% response rates.

What does the future hold for SLE patients?

Increasing understanding of the pathophysiology of SLE and the mechanisms involved are likely to move the management of SLE from 'empirical' to 'mechanistic'/'targeted' approach that has been recently discussed by several workers.[40-46] However, the availability of so many pathways would lead to the new therapeutic avenues or be the blind alleys?[41] Hundreds of stringently conducted clinical trials would have to be conducted without clear idea of which one is the most likely to yield a positive result. Should the target be a cell, a cytokine, a chemokine, an adipokine, an intracellular molecule in the signalling pathway? Should the target be the cell metabolism? Should it target any specific metabolic pathway (e.g. tryptophan pathway)? There is a glut of publications on different types of genetic, epigenetic, metabolic, cellular, subcellular abnormalities in lupus that could be targeted. Would it be a single (or limited number) target to control most of the SLE manifestations? Or, different targets for the protean manifestations of the disease would be required? It is going to be a difficult path to wade through but full of exciting possibilities. May be prolonged remissions and even drug-free remission in SLE could become possible. Wish I would be there to see these 'miracles'!

In conclusion, over the years, from being an uncommon esoteric disease, SLE has become one of the common conditions being seen, diagnosed and managed in most rheumatology–clinical immunology clinics around the country. Despite no 'specific' lupus drug being available (especially in India where even belimumab is not available), the management is generally satisfactory. However, the disease still remains an enigma due to its protean manifestations and unpredictable course. Yet, there is hope! Despite a number of heart-breaking results of randomized controlled trial of drugs that were expected to be block-busters, the future could not be that dismal with the possibility of the discovery of effective drugs for the different types and different complications/organ involvements seen in SLE.

REFERENCES

1. Wig KL. 'Memoirs of a Medical Man' 'ORIGINAL' Publishers: B2, Vardhaman Place, Nimri Commercial Centre, New Delhi 110052; Year 2000;107–114.
2. Mathews JD, Mackay IR, Whittingham S, Malcolm LA. Protein supplementation and enhanced antibody-producing capacity in New Guinean school-children. Lancet. 1972;30:675–7.
3. Aarden LA, de Groot ER, Feltkamp TE. Immunology of DNA. III. Crithidia luciliae, a simple substrate for the determination of anti-dsDNA with the immunofluorescence technique. Ann NY Acad Sci. 1975;254:505–15.

4. Avrameas S, Guilbert B. A method for quantitative determination of cellular immunoglobulins by enzyme-labeled antibodies. Eur J Immunol. 1971;1:394–6

5. Malaviya AN, Bhuyan UN, Kumar R, Baliga S. Connective tissue disorders in India I. Clinical and immurological profile of systemic lupus erythematosus. J Assoc Phy Ind. 1978;26:461–6.

6. Malaviya AN, Kar AK, Goswami S, Bhuyan UN, Kumar R, Malhotra KK, Taneja RL. Connective tissue disorders in India II. Clinical and immunological profile of Sjögren's syndrome. J Assoc Phy Ind. 1978;26:553–60.

7. Malaviya AN, Adhar GC, Pasricha JS. Connective tissue diseases in India III. Clinical and immunological profile of progressive systemic sclerosis. J Assoc Phy Ind. 1979;27:395–400.

8. Malaviya AN, Ahuja GK, Narayanan K, Dutt P. Connective tissue diseases in India IV. Clinical and immunological profile of polymyositis and dermatomyositis. J Assoc Phy Ind. 1981;29:309–14.

9. Malaviya AN, Narayanan K, Khan KM, Tiwari SC. Connective tissue diseases versus overlap syndrome. J Assoc Phy Ind. 1984;32:555–9.

10. Malaviya AN Zaidi Z. Connective tissue diseases in India VIII. Familial aggregation. J Assoc Phy Ind. 1984:32:793–7.

11. Malaviya AN, Singh RR, Kumar A. Systemic lupus erythematosus in northern India: A review of 329 cases. J Assoc Phy Ind. 1988;36:476–80.

12. Malaviya AN, Chandrasekaran AN, Kuamr A, Sharma PN. Occasional Series—lupus around the world: Systemic lupus erythematosus in India. Lupus. 1997;9:690–700.

13. Malaviya AN, Singh RR, Singh YN, Kapoor SK, Kumar A. Prevalence of systemic lupus erythematosus in India. Lupus. 1993;2:15–8.

14. Malaviya AN, Many A, Schwartz RS. Treatment of dermatomyositis with methotrexate. Lancet. 1968;291:465–8

15. Bhuyan U N, Malaviya AN. Antinuclear antibodies and pattern of nuclear immunofluorescence in systemic lupus erythematosus and other collagen vascular diseases. Ind J Med Res. 1976;64:895–902.

16. Bhuyan UN, Malaviya AN, Kumar, R, Malhotra KK, Tandon HD. Frequency and severity of renal lesions in systemic lupus erythematosus in north India. Ind J Med Res. 1977;66:965–73.

17. Chattopadhyay C, Malaviya AN, Uberoi S, Bhuyan UN, and Kumar R. Humoral and cell-mediated immune response in systemic lupus erythematosus. Ind J Med Res. 1977;64:220–6.

18. Narayanan K, Rajagopalan P, Malaviya AN. Immunospecificities of antinuclear antibodies in systemic connective tissue diseases in India. Ind J Med Res. 1983;77:87–95.

19. Malaviya AN, Khan KM, Tiwari SC, Bhuyan UN. Systemic connective tissue diseases in India VII. Deaths in systemic lupus erythematosus. J Assoc Phy Ind. 1984;32:313–6.

20. Malaviya AN, Misra R, Banerjee S, Kumar A, Tiwari SC, Bhuyan UN, Malhotra KK. Systemic lupus erythematosus in North Indian Asians; A prospective analysis of clinical and immunological features. Rheumatol Int. 1986;6:97–101.

21. Malaviya AN, Misra R, Kumar A, Tiwari SC. Systemic connective tissue diseases in India. IX. Survival in systemic lupus erythematosus. J Asso Phy Ind. 1987;35: 509–11.

22. Agarwal A, Singh RR, Kumar A, Misra R, Malaviya AN. Occurrence of systemic autoimmune disorders and autoantibodies in house-hold contacts of patients with systemic lupus erythematosus. Ind J Med Res. 1991; 94[B]:96–8.

23. Pande I, Sekharan NG, Kailash S, Uppal SS, Singh RR, Kumar A, Malaviya AN. Analysis of clinical and laboratory profile of Indian childhood systemic lupus erythematosus and its comparison with systemic lupus erythematosus in adults. Lupus. 1993;2:83–7.

24. Kumar A, Malaviya AN, Singh RR, Singh YN, Adya CM, Kakkar R. Survival of patients with systemic lupus erythematosus in India. Rheumatol Int. 1992;12:107–9.

25. Singh RR, Yen EY. SLE mortality remains disproportionately high, despite improvements over the last decade. Lupus. 2018; 25:727–34.

26. Ponticelli C, Moroni G. Hydroxychloroquine in systemic lupus erythematosus (SLE). Expert Opin Drug Saf. 2017;16:411–9.

27. Sousaa JR, Rosaa EPC, Nunesb IFdeOC, de-Carvalhob CMRG. Effect of vitamin D supplementation on patients with systemic lupus erythematosus: A systematic review. Revista Brasileira De Reumatologia. 2017;57(5):466–71.
28. Rho YH, Oeser A, Chung CP, Morrow JD, Stein CM. Drugs to treat systemic lupus erythematosus: Relationship between current use and cardiovascular risk factors. Arch Drug Info. 2008;1:23–28.
29. Chahal JS, Raina SK, Sharma KK, Kaur N. How common is Vitamin B12 deficiency—a report on deficiency among healthy adults from a medical college in rural area of North West India. Int J Nutr Pharmacol Neurolo Dis. 2014;4:241–6.
30. Malaviya AN, Mourou M. Should low-dose aspirin also be a background therapy for all patients with systemic lupus erythematosus (SLE)? Lupus. 2000;9:561–2.
31. Iudici M, Fasano S, Falcone GL, Pantano I, La-Montagna G1, Migliaresi S, et al. Low-dose aspirin as primary prophylaxis for cardiovascular events in systemic lupus erythematosus: A long-term retrospective cohort study. Rheumatology (Oxford). 2016;55:1623–30.
32. Galindo M, Gonzalo E, Martinez-Vidal MP, Montes S, Redondo N, Santiago B, et al. Immunohistochemical detection of intravascular platelet microthrombi in patients with lupus nephritis and anti-phospholipid antibodies. Rheumatology (Oxford). 2009;48,1003–1007.
33. Lee RZ, Hardiman O, O'Connell PG. Ibuprofen-induced meningoencephalitis. Rheumatology (Oxford). 2002;41:353–5.
34. Wallace DJ. Celecoxib for lupus. Arthritis Rheum. 2008;58:2923 (Letter).
35. Jorge AM, Lu N, Keller SF, Rai SK, Zhang Y, Choi HK. The effect of statin use on mortality in systemic autoimmune rheumatic diseases. J Rheumatol First Release September 1 2018.
36. McMahon M, Hahn BH, Skaggs BJ. Systemic lupus erythematosus and cardiovascular disease: prediction and potential for therapeutic intervention. Expert Rev Clin Immunol. 2011;7:227–41.
37. Sato EI. Methotrexate therapy in systemic lupus erythematosus. Lupus. 2001;10:162–4.
38. Sakthiswary R, Suresh E. Methotrexate in systemic lupus erythematosus: a systematic review of its efficacy. Lupus. 2014;23:225–35.
39. Davidson JE, Fu Q, Rao S, Magder LS, Petri M. Quantifying the burden of steroid-related damage in SLE in the Hopkins Lupus Cohort. Lupus Sci Med. 2018;5(1):e000237.
40. Thanou A, Merrill JT. Treatment of systemic lupus erythematosus: New therapeutic avenues and blind alleys. Nat Rev Rheumatol. 2014;10:23–34.
41. Touma Z, Gladman DD. Current and future therapies for SLE: obstacles and recommendations for the development of novel treatments. Lupus Science & Medicine. 2017;4:e000239;
42. Gatto M, Zen M, Iaccarino L, Doria A. New therapeutic strategies in systemic lupus erythematosus management. Arthritis Rheumatol. Published on-line on 11 December 2018.
43. Dorner T, Lipsky PE. Beyond pan-B-cell-directed therapy—new avenues and insights into the pathogenesis of SLE. Nat Rev Rheumatol. 2016;12:645–57.
44. Carreira PL, Isenberg DA. Recent developments in biologic therapies for the treatment of patients with systemic lupus erythematosus. Rheumatology (Oxford). 2018; pii: 4962137.
45. Sciascia S, Radin M, Roccatello D, Sanna G, Bertolaccini ML. Recent advances in the management of systemic lupus erythematosus. F1000Res. 2018 Jun 29;7:F1000 Faculty Rev-970.
46. Wallace DJ. The evolution of drug discovery in systemic lupus erythematosus. Nat Rev Rheumatol. 2015;11:616–20.

Pathogenesis of Lupus: Complex Interplay of Immunological Factors

Chengappa Kavadichanda G, Vir Singh Negi

INTRODUCTION

Systemic lupus erythematosus (SLE) is an enigma to both the treating physician and the scientist attempting to decipher the pathogenesis. The disease is thought to be a result of imbalance between the effector and regulatory arms of the immune system. The pathogenesis of SLE is complex with multiple players contributing to it. Lupus pathogenesis is a multistep process with genetic susceptibility to start with followed by a phase of preclinical lupus and then clinically manifest disease. This review presents the current evidence in a logical sequence to describe the interplay of immunological factors in the pathogenesis of lupus (Fig. 2.1).

GENETIC FACTORS

The role of genes in predisposing to SLE is reflected by twin and family studies. With a heritability of up to 43.9%, higher incidence in monozygotic twins (25–46%), a 5.87% relative risk among the first-degree relatives and a high-risk ratio of up to 29% in the siblings of SLE patients support the role of genes in disease pathogenesis. Further, the genes also modulate end organ involvement and severity of clinical manifestations in SLE.[1] Genes in the major histocompatibility complex (MHC) region play a major role in SLE susceptibility across various populations. With the advent of Genome Wide Association Studies (GWAS) numerous non MHC genes have also been implicated with SLE. A brief account of various HLA and non-HLA genes associated with SLE across various populations is represented in Tables 2.1 and 2.2.[2] Association of HLA with antibodies in SLE has been shown in Table 2.3 and the role of selected few genes are discussed later in the course of this review.

ENVIRONMENTAL FACTORS

Environmental exposure to various agents is the most important inciting event in initiating autoimmunity. Though epidemiological evidence for all the proposed toxins and infections are not convincing, *in vitro* data and animal models support such cause effect relationships (Table 2.4).[3]

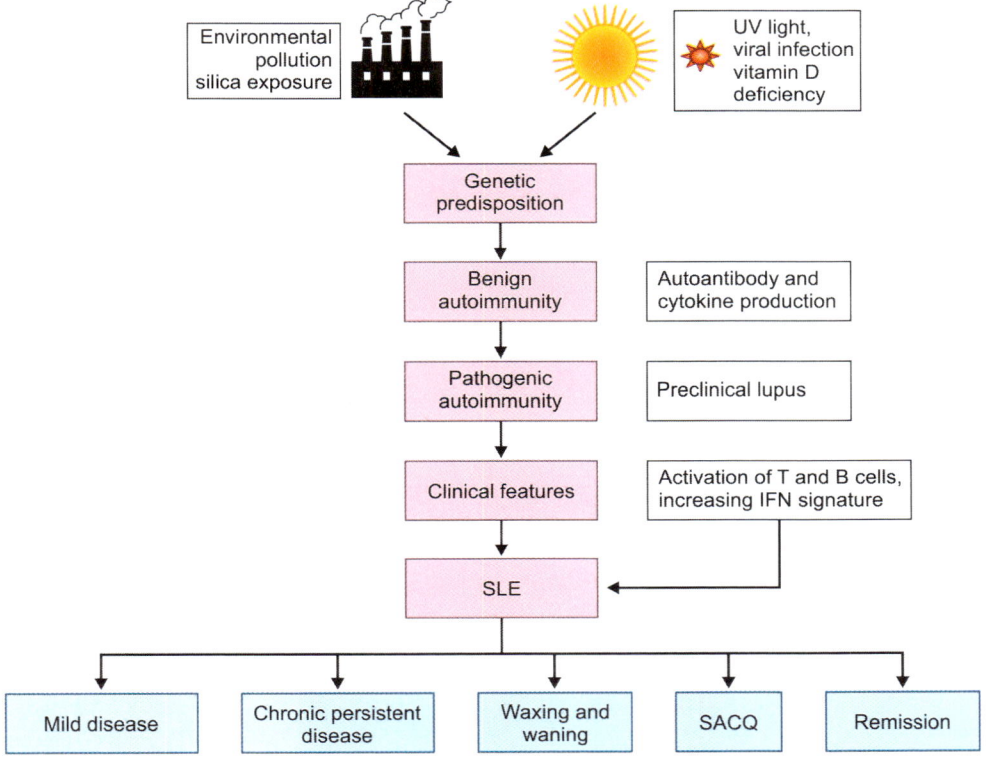

Fig. 2.1: Proposed model representing initiation and progress of systemic lupus erythematosus. UV—ultra-violet, IFN—interferon; SACQ—serologically active clinically quiescent

PRECLINICAL LUPUS

When genetically susceptible individuals are exposed to a variety of environmental factors, (Table 2.4) dysregulated activation of immune system occurs. The immune dysregulation which precedes autoantibody production progresses from a state of preclinical lupus to full blown SLE with end organ damage depending upon the persistence/magnitude of the environmental stimulus. The term preclinical is used for patients who have positive autoantibodies or clinical features insufficient for the classification of SLE. But lessons from animal studies and from autoantibody negative first-degree relatives of SLE patients have demonstrated immune aberrancies similar to that seen in SLE occurring years before autoantibody generation.[4]

STAGE OF IMMUNE DYSREGULATION PRIOR TO ANTIBODY GENERATION IN PRECLINICAL LUPUS

Lupus prone BXSB mouse models have demonstrated the role of interferons (IFN) secreted by plasmocytic dendritic cells (pDCs) as a chief driver of autoantibody generation. Depletion of pDCs in mice during the pre-autoantibody phase prevents rise in IFN levels resulting in hypogammaglobulinemia, decreased autoantibody generation and absence of kidney

Table 2.1: HLA and non-HLA genes associated with SLE across different population studies[2]

Gene function	Population			
	Asians	*Europeans*	*African*	*Hispanic Americans*
Antigen presentation	HLA-DR2, HLA-DR-3 HLA-DRB1*15:01 HLA-DRB1*15:02 HLA-DQA2	HLA-A1,HLA-DRB1*03:01B8, DR3, and DQ2	DRB1*15:03 and HLA-DRB1*08	HLA-DQA1, HLA-DQA2
Role in NFkB signalling	TNAIP1, TNFAIP3, SLC15A4,UBE2L3, HIC2, IRAK1	IKBKE,UBASH3A, TNAIP1, TNFAIP3, UBE2L3, HIC2, IRAK1	TNAIP1, TNFAIP3	IRAK1
Role in apoptosis and/or clearance of debris	IL-2/IL-21, ATG5, ITGAM,DNAse 1, ACP5/TRAP	Complement genes, IL-2/IL-21,ATG5, ITGAM, ACP5/TRAP	IL-2/IL-21	ITGAM
Role in TLR and interferon signalling	STAT4, RASGRP3, IRF5/TNPO3, TLR7	IFIH1, STAT4, PRDM1, IRF5/TNPO3, IRF7, IRF8, TLR7	STAT4, IRF5/ TNPO3,IRF7	STAT4, IRF5/TNPO3
Role in cellular growth and adhesion and endocytosis	TNXB, HIP1	UHRF1BP1	-	-
Role in B cell immunity	NCF2, IL-10, BANK1, BLK, ELF1	NCF2, IL-10, BANK1, BLK, IKZF3, CD 40	IL-10, BANK1, BLK, IKZF3	BANK1, BLK, IKZF3
Role in T cell immunity	TNFSF4, IKZF1, AFF, ETS1	PTPN22, TNFSF4, IKZF1, CSK, TYK2, SH2D1A, CD44, PHHX	-	PTPN22, TNFSF4

Table 2.2: Genetic associations of SLE reported from India

Associated with SLE susceptibility[37–42]	*Associated with development of lupus nephritis*[42–45]	*Associated with development of medium vessel vasculitis*[46]
CTLA 4, FCG3A F/V 176, TLR 9, IL1Ra, DNAse 1	C1q heterozygous C to T [rs121909581] in exon 2	MBL codon 54 rs1800450 IL-1β (-511 C/T) polymorphism
Vitamin D receptor FokI (Ff) and TaqI (Tt) heterozygotes), IL-6-174 G>C polymorphism, TNF-α and LTα gene polymorphisms	DNASE1 A / G (rs1053874) in exon 8 IL-1β (-511 C/T)polymorphism TNF-α and LTα gene polymorphisms MCP-1 (-2518A/G) polymorphism	

inflammation. Further, administration of IFN type I/II receptor antagonist prevents autoantibody generation in young MRL-Fas[lpr] mice. Though there are evidence supporting the development of autoantibodies independent of pDCs and IFN, IFN pathway still is the most important initiation pathway in precipitation of autoimmunity.[5] Similar findings of increase in IFN type I, interferon gamma-induced protein 10 (IP-10) and elevated IFN

Table 2.3: HLA-autoantibody association in SLE

HLA class II allele	Associated antibodies
HLA-DR2/DX	Anti-Sm
HLA-DR3/DX, DQ2	Anti-Ro and Anti-La
HLA-DR2/DR3	Anti-Ro, Anti-La, Anti-Sm, Anti-dsDNA
HLA-DR3/DR3	Anti-Sm
HLA-DR4/DQ8	Anti-cardiolipin, lupus anticoagulant, anti-β2 glycoprotein I
HLA-DR4	Anti-Sm, anti-RNP
HLA-DR5	Absence of anti-Sm and anti-RNP

Table 2.4: Proposed roles of environmental factors in development of SLE

Environmental factor	Evidence for disease development	Mechanism
Respirable silica dust (crystalline quartz)	Dose response relationship of silica exposure and increase SLE risk in various populations Exacerbates lupus in murine models, increases levels of serum auto-antibodies, immune complexes, glomerulonephritis and proteinuria	Behaves as an immune adjuvant, apoptosis induction and release of intracellular antigenscytokines Increasing pro-inflammatory oxidative stress and T cell responses
High-level exposure to dusts (World Trade Center disaster)	Rates of composite systemic autoimmune diseases was high in workers exposed to the highest levels	Acute high dose dust exposure can lead to pulmonary inflammation, oxidative stress and epigenetic changes
Particulate air pollution	Overall evidence of increased incidence of systemic autoimmune diseases	Possibly similar to silica and acute dust exposure
Cigarette smoking (tars, nicotine, carbon monoxide, polycyclic aromatic hydrocarbons and free radicals)	Meta-analysis of studies of smoking and SLE risk → Current smokers had a modestly elevated SLE risk (OR 1.5; 95% CI 1.09, 2.08) compared to non-smokers Evidence from Nurses' Health Study prospective cohorts: Current, smoking was strongly related to the risk of anti-double stranded DNA-positive subtype of SLE (1.86; 95% CI 1.14, 3.04])	Induce oxidative stress leading to genetic and epigenetic mutations Stimulates the expression of CD95 on B and CD4 on T cell surfaces-inducing autoimmunity Overall increase in pro-inflammatory cytokines
Solvents (e.g. dry cleaning solvents, nail polish removers, paints, perfumes)	Contradicting results with some studies showing positive and a few other studies showing no association with exposure and development of SLE.	May affect oxidative stress and/or sex hormone homeostasis
Pesticide exposure Heavy metals	Inconclusive evidence Association of SLE with residential proximity to a uranium processing plant	Behaves as an immune adjuvant

(Contd...)

Table 2.4: Proposed roles of environmental factors in development of SLE (*Contd...*)

Environmental factor	Evidence for disease development	Mechanism
	Higher prevalence of ANA in Mercury-exposed gold miners *In vitro* studies using mononuclear cells (PBMC) from healthy donors have shown evidence of increased proinflammatory cytokine release on treatment with inorganic mercury (iHg). Development of autoimmunity in genetically predisposed animal models when exposed to both inorganic and organic mercury	Apoptosis induction and release of intracellular antigens Increasing pro-inflammatory cytokines, oxidative stress and T cell responses
Ultra-violet exposure	Inconclusive evidence Clinical experience shows systemic disease flare associated to prolonged sunlight exposure	UV-B radiation results in induction of reactive oxygen species, leading to DNA damage, production of novel forms of autoantigens and autoreactive T cells, and may have immunomodulatory effects on T cells and cytokines
Vitamin D deficiency	Deficient levels have been found across various autoimmune diseases. Few unconvincing studies have demonstrated improvement ion disease activity with vitamin D supplementation	Vitamin D 1,25 (OH)2D3, acts plays a major role in increasing T regs and decreasing the inflammatory phenotype of T lymphocytes
Chronic infections, EBV and parvovirus B19 infections	Meta-analysis of twenty-five case control studies demonstrated a statistically significant higher seroprevalence of EBV anti-viral capsid antigen IgG (OR 2.08, 95% CI 1.15 to 3.76, p = 0.007) and antibodies to EBV early antigen diffuse, a marker of viral replication, in patients with *existing SLE* patients compared to normal individuals (OR 4.5; 95% CI 3.00 to 11.06, p <0.00001) High chances of publication bias in this paper	Molecular mimicry, chronic activation of the effector arm of immune system By-stander activation of innate and adaptive immune cells

signatures are also demonstrated prior to increase in the levels of various autoantibodies in humans.[6]

Recent data suggests increase in IFN type II (IFN-γ) level prior to IFN type I level, implicating IFN-γ as the primary driver of IFN I response. Elevated IFN-γ along with chemokines IP-10 and MCP-3 levels precedes elevation in IFN-α and autoantibodies in the serum among individuals prone to develop SLE.[7] The major sources of IFN-γ are the T cells and natural killer (NK) cells. The NK cells play a dual role in mediation and regulation of inflammation in SLE. A subset of these cells have features of dendritic cells and may be responsible for increased production of IFN.[8] This is also complemented by abnormal Th2 activation and release of IL-4,5 and 6 occurring approximately 3 years prior to autoantibody production in genetically predisposed patients.[9] Over all, the current evidence supports a model where in initial environmental trigger upregulates IFN-γ, Th1 and Th2 cytokines, which drives IFN-α production, B cell activation, ultimately resulting in variable autoimmunity.

STAGE OF EARLY AUTOANTIBODY FORMATION

The autoantibodies in SLE appear approximately 9.4 years (mean 3.3 years) prior to clinical signs or symptoms. Various autoantibodies starting with anti-nuclear antibody (ANA) and anti-Ro progressing to anti-cardiolipin (aCL) and anti-Smith (Sm) appear at different time frames during the course of immune dysregulation. The order of appearance of these antibodies have no bearing on the outcome and prognosis of SLE. Current evidence suggests that a marked rise in the titer of anti-dsDNA antibodies may herald the onset of SLE in asymptomatic individuals.[3]

PROGRESS OF AUTOANTIBODIES: FROM BENIGN TO PATHOGENIC

The autoantibodies seen in SLE are generated against various cellular components like DNA, DNA binding proteins, RNA, RNA-binding proteins, ribonuclear proteins and phospholipids in the cell membrane. The primary autoantibodies generated are of IgM subclass which are either pathogenic or protective. Some of the natural IgM autoantibodies have anti-apoptotic, and inhibitory effect on TLR mediated cell activation.[10] However, as the immune dysregulation progresses, the autoantibodies undergo class switch to IgG, IgA or IgE subtype and escape into the intravascular or mucosal surface and get deposited in various organs.

Some of the ANAs also act as DAMPs and upregulates inflammatory pathways. Antibody production in SLE is further enhanced by elevated IL-21 and T follicular (Tfh) cell activation. In addition, excessive B cell stimulation by antigen primed CD4+ helper cells and B cell activating factors (BAFF and APRIL) also increases antibody production. The specific autoantibodies in SLE like the anti-Sm and anti-dsDNA are used as markers of diagnosis. Autoantibodies against C1q, dsDNA, anti-Ribosomal P play important roles in the pathogenesis by getting deposited in renal and neural tissues[11] leading to amplification of inflammatory cascade.

ROLE OF DEFECTIVE APOPTOSIS, COMPLEMENTS, CELL DEBRIS CLEARANCE AND PAMPS

Various factors including toxins, infections, physical and psychological stress lead to increased apoptosis of cells which in normal individuals are effectively cleared by phagocytes. Several GWAS studies in SLE have shown strong association with genes affecting the receptors responsible for clearance of cell debris and immune complexes (FCGR2A, FCGR2B, FCGR3B, ATG5, CLEC16A). This is further compounded by an intrinsic defect in macrophages to effectively phagocytose cell debris in SLE.

Clearance of immune complexes and debris is naturally aided via coating of apoptotic cells with C1q complement component, C-reactive proteins (CRP) or serum amyloid P (SAP).[12,13] Low complement levels, defective complement receptors and antibodies to complement components (e.g. anti-C1q) result in poor immune complex handling and thus favours deposition in tissues. These defects also lead to persistence of the self and foreign antigens resulting in excessive DAMP-mediated toll-like receptors (TLR) stimulation.[14]

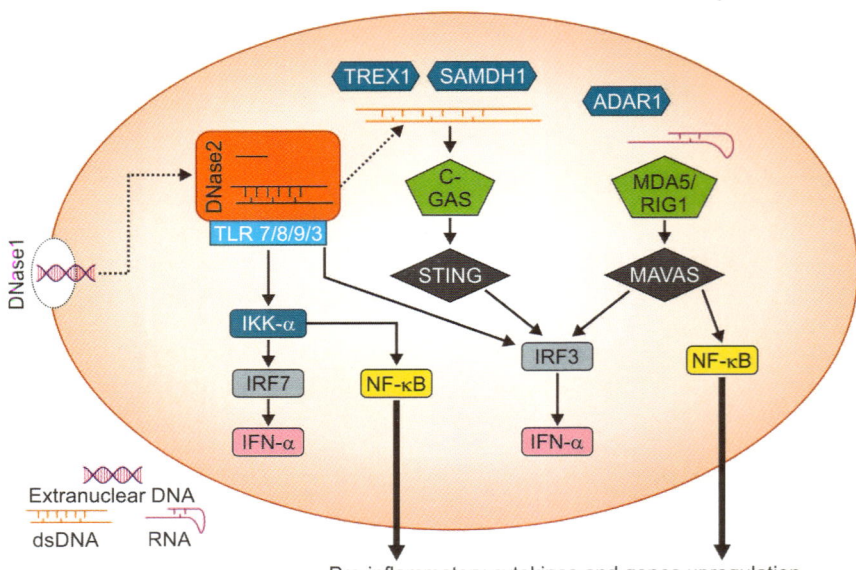

Fig. 2.2: Nucleic acid sensors and their role in inflammation. DNase 1 and 2 are enzymes that degrade extracellular and endosomal chromatin debris. Their low levels in SLE may lead to persistence of nuclear material. They are ligands for toll-like receptors (TLRs), C-GAS STING, RIG-1 MAVAS and upregulate interferon I and NF-κB mediated pro-inflammatory cytokine production

Toll-like receptors are one of the major driver of innate immune pathways and are implicated in several autoimmune diseases including SLE. While TLRs 3, 7, 8 detects RNA, the TLR 9 detects CpG DNA. Genetic defects, upregulation, and aberrant activation of these TLRs are identified across various organs involved in SLE. The recruitment of TLRs causes IFN production and NFkB-mediated upregulation of inflammation. Besides the TLRs, various other intracytoplasmic nucleic acid sensors like MDA-5, MVAS and c-GAS also play a role in induction of type I IFN (Fig. 2.2). The role of components involved in the downstream pathway of these PAMPs like the STAT, TYK2 and others in SLE are summarized in Table 2.5.

Besides this DNase I, the enzyme responsible for the degradation of extracellular chromatin material released by dying cells are also reported to be deficient in SLE. The persistent chromatin material or other debris are endocytosed by dendritic cells (DC) activating the endosomal TLRs and other pattern recognition receptor (PRR) (Fig. 2.2) leading to the upregulation of inflammatory cascade.

CONTRIBUTION OF CYTOKINES IN SLE

Cytokines are amongst the most important soluble mediators responsible for cross talk between cells. Evidence from lupus studies shows elevation of both the pro and anti-inflammatory cytokines. Tumour necrosis factor (TNF), interleukins (IL) 4, 6 and 10 along with type I and II interferons are found in higher levels in patients with SLE as compared to healthy subjects.

Recently, IL-17/23 axis as well as relative IL-2 deficiency is being increasingly implicated in SLE.[15] IL-2 has a major role in maintaining T-reg cell numbers and function. It restricts

Table 2.5: Role of pattern recognition receptors and their downstream signalling molecules in SLE

Pattern recognition receptor	Location	Function
Toll-like receptors		
TLR3	Endosome	dsRNA sensing and type I IFN induction
TLR7/8	Endosome	ssRNA sensing and type I IFN induction
TLR9	Endosome	Cpg DNA sensor and type I IFN
PTPN22	Cytoplasm	Negative regulator of TLR signaling
IRAK1/ IRF 3,5,7,8	Cytoplasm	Downstream mediators for TLR
IKBE	Cytoplasm	Downstream mediators for TLR
Other PAMPs and downstream molecules		
STING	Cytoplasm	DNA sensor and type I IFN inducer
MDA5	Cytoplasm	Cytosolic dsRNA sensor and IFN I inducer
TYK2	Cytoplasm (components of receptor downstream signals)	IFNAR signaling
STAT4	Cytoplasm (Components of receptor downstream signals)	IFNAR signaling
ITGAM	Cytoplasm	Enhancer of phagocytosis

the expression of IL-17, which is an important pro-inflammatory cytokine released by the Th17 cells. Thought the precise role of IL-17 in immune dysregulation in SLE is not known, urinary biomarker studies have shown increased expression of Th17-related genes in active lupus nephritis (LN).[16] The efficacy of ustekinumab, IL-12/IL-23 p40 antagonist in various animal models and a phase 2 study in humans further implicates the IL-23/IL-17 pathway in the immunopathogenesis of lupus.[17]

CONTRIBUTION OF INTERFERONS IN SLE

IFN-α, a type I IFN is released by the innate cells and plasmacytoid dendritic cells (pDC) in response to viral infections or self-antigens.[1] IFN-α results in upregulation of adaptive immunity by increased B cell survival due to induction of B cell activating factor (BAFF) and A proliferation-inducing ligand (APRIL). They have a pleotropic effect on various immune cells (Fig. 2.3). The role of IFN-α in SLE is further reflected by the high IFN-α signature in patients with active lupus nephritis and the promising efficacy of various IFN-α antagonists in the treatment of lupus.[18] Various IFN-α response proteins, like IP-10, SIGLEC1 (CD169) and CD64, are being explores as biomarkers for lupus activity.

DEFECTS IN CELLULAR COMPONENTS OF INNATE IMMUNE SYSTEM

Neutrophils

Neutrophils make-up the largest compartment of leucocytes in adults and are the first line of defense in any immune response. They are responsible for sequestering and eliminating foreign or self-elements by means of phagocytosis and production of reactive oxygen species. The neutrophils also release alarmins, proinflammatory cytokines, and various proteolytic enzymes stored in their cytoplasmic granules. These cells are responsible for clearing and trapping foreign bodies by forming 'neutrophils extracellular traps' (NETs).

Neutrophils in SLE have several functional and phenotypic abnormalities and have an important role in inflammation, autoantibody production, organ damage and determining prognosis.

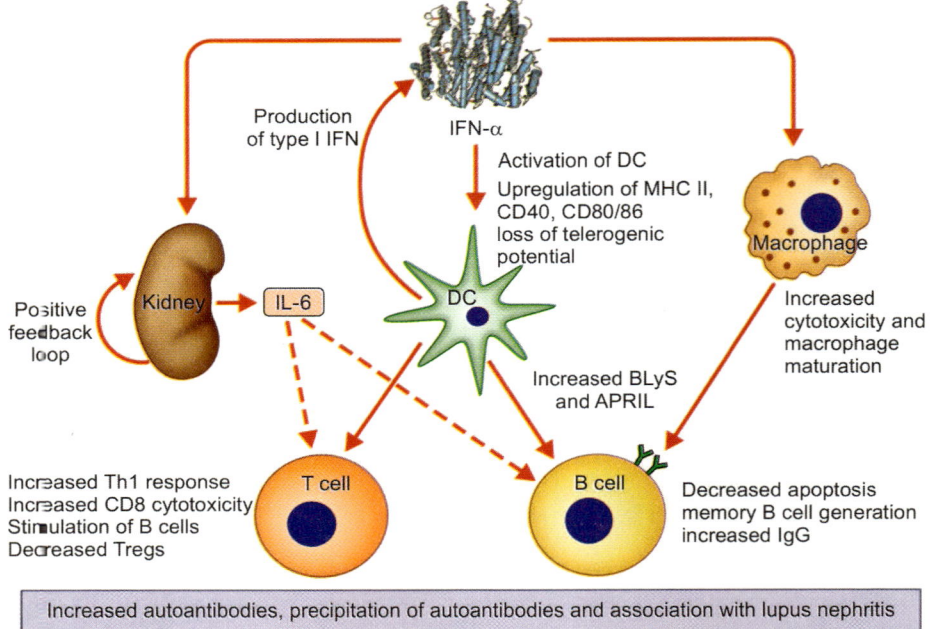

Fig. 2.3: Role of IFN-alpha in SLE immunopathogenesis (solid arrows—direct effect, dotted arrows—indirect effect). APRIL—a proliferation inducing ligand, BLyS—B lymphocyte stimulator

Low Density Granulocytes (LDG)

Neutrophil subsets in SLE have a lesser density, similar to that of monocytes but express the surface markers similar to neutrophils. The LDGs have an immature nuclear morphology and have a propensity to produce higher levels of TNF, IFN I and II, damage endothelium and form NETs.[19] Thought the pathological role of LGDs is not confirmed in SLE, the propensity of these cells to push the immune response into overdrive has generated a lot of research interest on these cells.

NETosis

NETosis is a form of neutrophil cell death characterized by the release of chromatin material and antimicrobial peptide into the extracellular space. The steps involved in forming NETs and its role in SLE is represented in Fig. 2.4.[20] NETosis is implicated in the pathophysiology of SLE as it results in amplification of cytokine release (chiefly TNF, IL-17 and IFN) and in prolonging exposure of autoantigens making them targets for autoantibody formation.

Monocytes and Macrophages

Monocytes are derived from myeloid cell lines and either stay as circulating monocytes or transform into tissue macrophages. Naïve (M0) macrophages from the bone marrow polarises to either the classical M1 or alternative M2 phenotype based on the effect of polarising cytokines on them. The M1 macrophages are considered to be inflammatory and the M2 are responsible for wound healing, angiogenesis, resolution of inflammation and fibrosis.

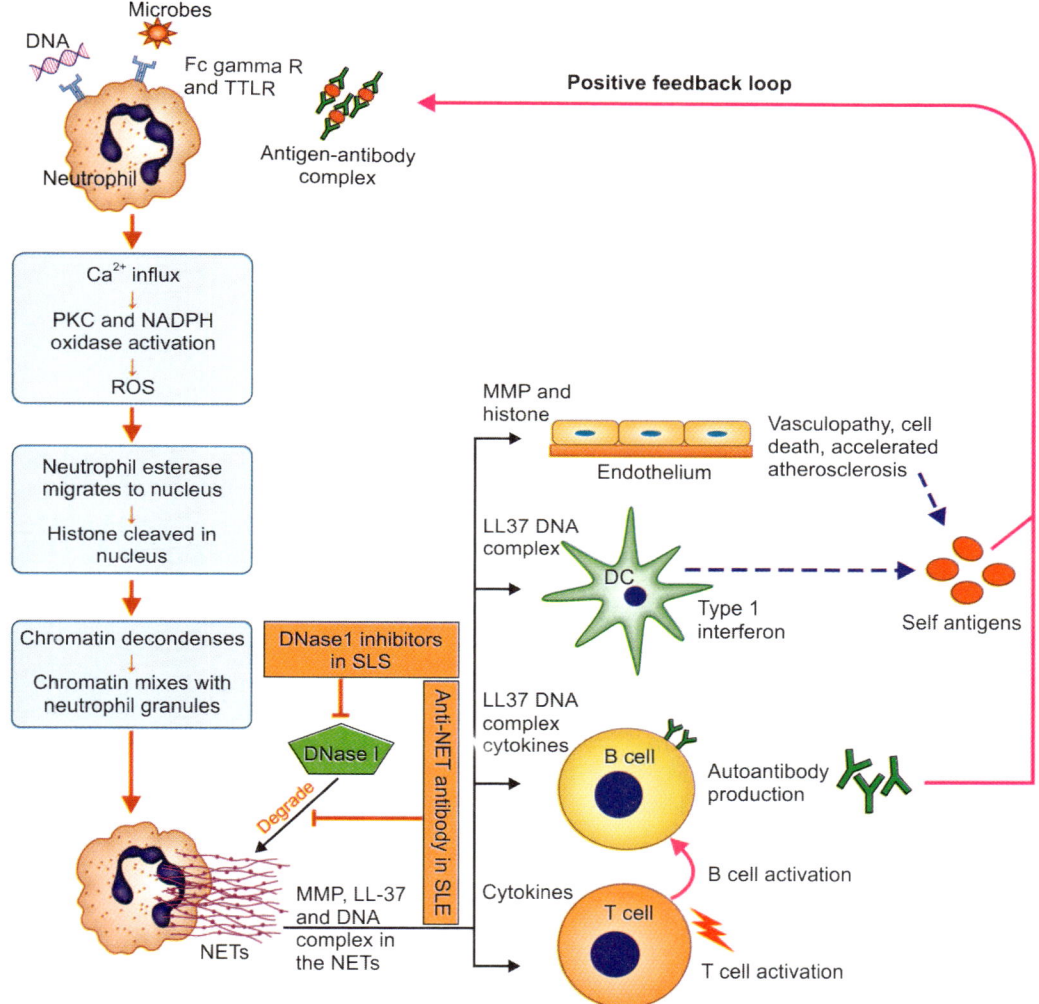

Fig. 2.4: Neutrophil extracellular traps (NETosis) and SLE. MMP—matrix metalloproteinase; PKC—protein kinase C; ROS—reactive oxygen species

M1 macrophages when activated by PAMPs like the lipopolysaccharide in the presence of IFN increasingly expresses monocyte chemoattractant protein 1 (MCP 1) which is amplified in SLE.[21] Activated macrophages have an increased propensity to release cytokines and present autoantigens to T cells. The role of monocytes, predominantly the M2 phenotype in damaging glomeruli and the vessel endothelium has been elucidated and the presence of such monocytes in renal tissue is associated with poorer outcomes in lupus nephritis.[22]

Dendritic Cells

Dendritic cells (DC) are responsible for processing antigens and presenting them to T cells thus bridging innate with adaptive immune system. They are classified into myeloid DC (classical DC), plasmacytoid DC (pDC), monocyte associated DC and tissue specific DC.

DC are responsible for effective clearance of apoptotic debris by the means of various receptors. This step is compromised in patients prone to develop lupus leading to prolonged self-antigen exposure, resulting in disruption of immune tolerance. The pDCs are a major source of type I IFN which plays an important role in initiation and amplification of immune dysregulation.[23]

T Cells

All the main T cell subsets (CD4+, CD8+, and double negative T cells) are aberrantly activated in SLE. This results in inappropriate cytokine release and excessive activation of B cells. Several alterations are noted in the T cell receptors (TCRs) and the downstream signaling of these cells in patients with lupus (Fig. 2.5).

T follicular helper cells (Tfh) are required for immunoglobulin class switching, formation of memory B cells and determining the clonality of B cells with the help of IL-21. The Tfh cells express CXCR5 which allows them to localise to B cell zone in the follicle. Their functions are regulated by the expression of programmed cell death protein 1 (PD-1) which is a negative regulator, the inducible T-cell co-stimulator (ICOS) and the OX40 ligand which are positive regulators. Studies involving lupus mice models have demonstrated overexpression of ICOS and OX 40 on the Tfh cells. In human studies, Tfh cells are increased both in the tertiary lymphoid organs (TLOs) and in circulation (cTfh). The role played by Tfh in the pathogenesis of SLE and the various factors influencing Tfh activation is represented in Fig. 2.5.[24]

Th17 cells are emerging as novel players in lupus pathogenesis. Th 17 cells are activated by IL-23 and they produce various IL-17 cytokines (IL-17A to IL-17F). The level of these cytokines, mainly the IL17A corelates with disease activity in lupus. Studies from lupus mouse models and humans have demonstrated an increase in the numbers of Th17 in patients with SLE as compared to healthy controls.[25] These cells are also found in tissue biopsies of kidneys in LN, reflecting a local as well as a systemic role in immune dysregulation. Activation of the Th17 cells tilts the balance of Th17/T-reg towards a Th17 predominant inflammatory phenotype.[26]

B Cells

The production of autoantibodies, mainly against the self-nuclear antigens represents the loss of tolerance in B cells. B cell related gene (BLK, BANK and PTPN22) polymorphism have been associated with the development of aberrant response to autoantigens. Beyond antibody production B cells also double up as antigen presenting cells and a source of inflammatory cytokines. The B lymphocytes are activated by different cells including the Th1, Tfh, and are affected by NETosis (Figs 2.3–2.5). B-cells can also activate the TLRs on the innate cells by producing high affinity antibodies against chromatin materials resulting in an antigen antibody complex. These complexes also activates the classical complement pathway, resulting in damage of tissues and further precipitation of NETosis. Autoantibody subclasses IgG and IgM are usually implicated in the pathogenesis of SLE. Recent evidence however has demonstrated a high level of IgE and IgE subclass of autoantibodies along with activated basophils in patients with lupus.[27] Experiments in mouse models have demonstrated a beneficial effect of IgE depletion in treating renal disease, thus throwing open a new vista for possible experimental therapeutic intervention.[28] Several therapeutic trials with rituximab (anti-CD20), belimumab (anti-BAFF) and tabalumab (anti-APRIL) though not completely successful have indirectly demonstrated the role of B cells in the pathophysiology of SLE.[29]

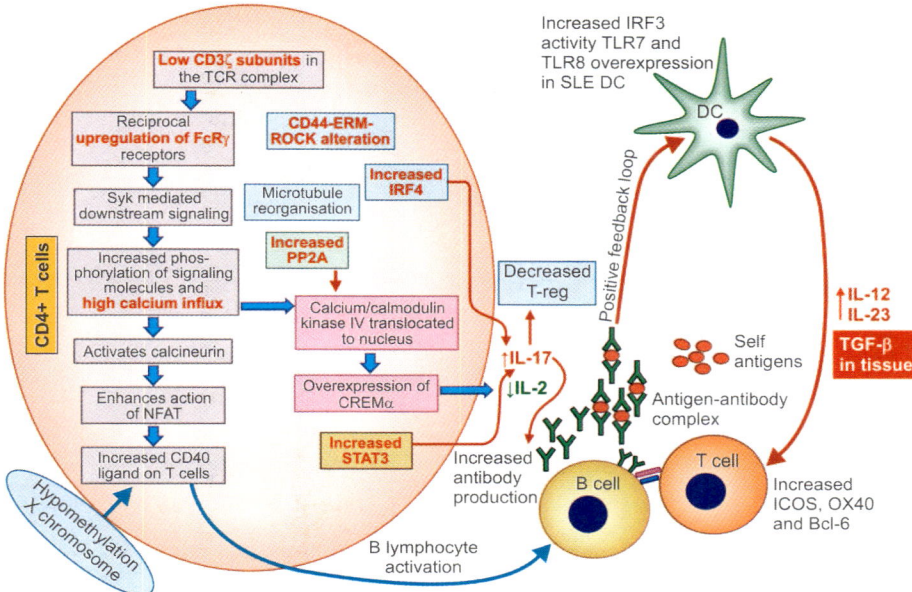

Fig. 2.5: Innate defects in T cells (highlighted in red with black background) and their interaction with various immune cells in SLE pathophysiology. CREM—cAMP response element modulator; ERM—ezrin/radixin/moesin protein complex; ICOS—inducible T-cell co-stimulator; IRF—Interferon regulatory factor; NFAT—nuclear factor of activated T cells; PP2—protein phosphate 2; Rho-associated protein kinase (ROCK); Syk—spleen tyrosine kinase; TCR—T cell receptor

Regulatory Cells

Regulatory cell are the components of the immune system that form the anti-inflammatory arm. The regulatory cell population predominantly comprises of T and B regulatory cells (T-reg, B-reg).

T Regulatory Cells

Data on the number and function of T-reg cells in SLE is inconsistent probably due to the choice of cell surface markers used in detecting the T-regs and the different disease states during the time of analysis. T-regs and Th17 cells have high plasticity and a tendency to convert to the former or latter cell type depending on the cytokine milieu. SLE has low IL-2 due to cyclic AMP response element modulator alpha (CREMα) overexpression and upregulation of calcium/calmodulin-dependent kinase IV (CaMK4) (Fig. 2.5). These changes along with high levels of IFN, TNF and IL-17 cytokines makes T-regs reduce their FoxP3 expression and become ex-T-reg cells. This phenotype characterizes inflammatory T-regs. The role of IL-2 deficiency and T-regs is further supported by the therapeutic trials involving low dose IL-2 injections in patients with SLE and resultant increase in the T-reg numbers and decrease in SLE disease activity.[30]

B Regulatory Cells

B10 cells are the best characterized and widely studied subtype of regulatory B cells. The main function of B-reg is production of IL-10. In human SLE there is an increase in B-reg

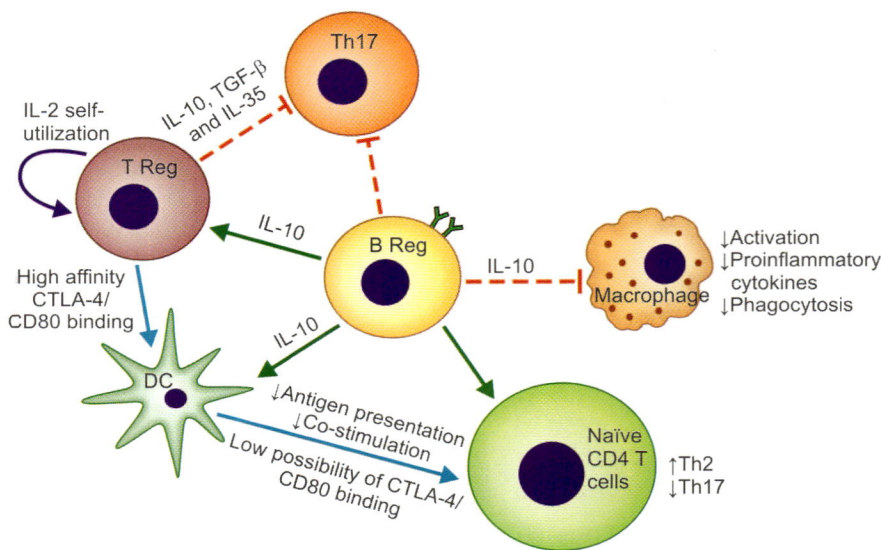

Fig. 2.6: Regulatory system in SLE. Broken red line—negative regulation, green arrow—positive effect, blue line—indirect effect of T-regs on T cells

numbers which negatively corelates with autoantibody titres and disease activity. There is also emerging evidence of a functional defects of B-reg in SLE.[31] The interaction between various regulatory cells, and effector immune cells is represented in Fig. 2.6.

END RESULT OF IMMUNE ABERRANCIES: END-ORGAN MANIFESTATION

Lupus is diagnosed on the basis of the end-organ involvement. All the discussed immune aberrancies orchestrate to culminate to involve different organs.

Renal Involvement

Lupus nephritis is proposed to start with the deposition of immune complexes (IC) on the glomerular basement membrane (GBM) due to the fenestrations in the capillary endothelium and the cationic nature of the glomeruli. The deposition of ICs on the GBM triggers the activation of the classical complement pathway. Components (C3a and C5a) of complement activation acts as attractants to a variety of cells including the neutrophils. The natural process of clearance of these immune complexes opsonized by complements is impaired in SLE due to either a deficiency in complements or defects in various receptors like FcγR. The combination of increased neutrophil chemotaxis with uncleared ICs precipitates NET formation and damage of endothelium by reactive oxygen species resulting in local amplification of the inflammatory loop.

The recurrent bouts of such inflammatory insults in the tissue leads to differentiation of M0 macrophages to predominantly M1 phenotype. This is then followed by infiltration of various immune cells of Th1,Th2, Th17, and B cells thus perpetuating a chronic inflammatory state. Besides the classically accepted IC model, the renal resident cells like the podocytes, pericytes and tubular cells also play major roles in determining inflammation and treatment response.

Cutaneous Involvement

Various triggers like UV-B radiation activate keratinocytes and increases production of IFN-I, various chemokines and precipitates cell death. Excess of nuclear chromatin and other intracellular antigens are exposed to the periphery initiating immune complex formation.[32] Once the formation of ICs occurs, the immune system follows a similar course as seen in kidney.

Neuropsychiatric Lupus (NPSLE)

Neuropsychiatric SLE is the least understood end-organ manifestation in lupus given the difficulty in obtaining the affected tissues and absence of reliable biomarkers for analysis. Inflammation of CNS is evidenced by the demonstration of high levels of inflammatory cytokines in the CSF and serum of the patients with NPSLE. The factors in the serum enter the brain parenchyma due to leakage of the blood brain barrier (BBB) and blood CSF barrier (BCSFB).[33] Though the reason for disruption of these barriers is not clear, experimental evidence from animal models have shown that endothelial changes in the blood vessels of brain could be the potential first step. Autoantibodies like anti-ribosomal P antibody[34] and anti-N-methyl-D-aspartate receptor (NMDAR)[35] antibodies along with other ICs and complement activation alter the NFkB-mediated inflammation and cell adhesion molecules (ICAM)[36] on the endothelium. This breach in the barrier is confirmed by the demonstration of various brain-specific and non-specific autoantibodies in both the serum and CSF of patients of NPSLE.

Various autoantibodies including the anti-dsDNA, anti-Ribo P, anti-cardiolipin, anti-NMDAR antibodies cause neuronal and glial apoptosis. They also play a role in synapse pruning, IC deposition and complement activation in the brain parenchyma. All this together leads to either a focal vascular pathology like stroke, focal demyelination, vasculitis or a diffuse pathology like psychosis, depression, mood disorder, movement disorder or seizures.

CONCLUSION

Though the pathogenesis of SLE is extremely complex, we have come a long way since the description of LE cell phenomenon in 1948 and optimistically the research seems to be moving in the right direction. The current understanding of the disease has resulted in the developments of a range of targeted drugs undergoing trials for the treatment of SLE. This enthusiastic upswing in treatment strategy targeting specific immune imbalance has encouraged rheumatologists to contemplate 'treat to target' concepts in the management of SLE.

REFERENCES

1. Tsokos GC, Lo MS, Costa Reis P, Sullivan KE. New insights into the immunopathogenesis of systemic lupus erythematosus. Nat Rev Rheumatol. 2016 22;12(12):716–30.
2. James JA. Clinical Perspectives on Lupus Genetics: Advances and Opportunities. Rheum Dis Clin North Am. 2014 Aug;40(3):413–32.
3. Parks CG, de Souza Espindola Santos A, Barbhaiya M, Costenbader KH. Understanding the role of environmental factors in the development of systemic lupus erythematosus. Best Pract Res Clin Rheumatol. 2017 Jun;31(3):306–20.
4. Robertson JM, James JA. Preclinical SLE. Rheum Dis Clin North Am. 2014 Nov;40(4):621–35.
5. Huang X, Dorta-Estremera S, Yao Y, Shen N, Cao W. Predominant role of plasmacytoid dendritic cells in stimulating systemic autoimmunity. Front Immunol. 2015 Oct 12;6:526.

6. Eriksson C, Rantapää-Dahlqvist S. Cytokines in relation to autoantibodies before onset of symptoms for systemic lupus erythematosus. Lupus. 2014 Jun;23(7):691–6.

7. Munroe ME, Lu R, Zhao YD, Fife DA, Robertson JM, Guthridge JM, et al. Altered type II interferon precedes autoantibody accrual and elevated type I interferon activity prior to systemic lupus erythematosus classification. Ann Rheum Dis. 2016 Nov;75(11):2014–21.

8. Cruz-González D de J, Gómez-Martin D, Layseca-Espinosa E, Baranda L, Abud-Mendoza C, Alcocer-Varela J, et al. Analysis of the regulatory function of natural killer cells from patients with systemic lupus erythematosus. Clin Exp Immunol. 2018 Mar;191(3):288–300.

9. Lu R, Munroe ME, Guthridge JM, Bean KM, Fife DA, Chen H, et al. Dysregulation of innate and adaptive serum mediators precedes systemic lupus erythematosus classification and improves prognostic accuracy of autoantibodies. J Autoimmun. 2016 Nov;74:182–93.

10. Chen Y, Khanna S, Goodyear CS, Park YB, Raz E, Thiel S, et al. Regulation of dendritic cells and macrophages by an anti-apoptotic cell natural antibody that suppresses TLR responses and inhibits inflammatory arthritis. J Immunol Baltim Md 1950. 2009 Jul 15;183(2):1346–59.

11. DeGiorgio LA, Konstantinov KN, Lee SC, Hardin JA, Volpe BT, Diamond B. A subset of lupus anti-DNA antibodies cross-reacts with the NR2 glutamate receptor in systemic lupus erythematosus. Nat Med. 2001 Nov;7(11):1189–93.

12. Lleo A, Selmi C, Invernizzi P, Podda M, Gershwin ME. The consequences of apoptosis in autoimmunity. J Autoimmun. 2008 Nov;31(3):257–62.

13. Truedsson L, Bengtsson AA, Sturfelt G. Complement deficiencies and systemic lupus erythematosus. Autoimmunity. 2007 Jan 1;40(8):560–6.

14. Rose T, Dörner T. Drivers of the immunopathogenesis in systemic lupus erythematosus. Best Pract Res Clin Rheumatol. 2017;31(3):321–33.

15. Oke V, Brauner S, Larsson A, Gustafsson J, Zickert A, Gunnarsson I, et al. IFN-λ1 with Th17 axis cytokines and IFN-α define different subsets in systemic lupus erythematosus (SLE). Arthritis Res Ther. 2017 15;19(1):139.

16. Kwan BC-H, Tam L-S, Lai K-B, Lai FM-M, Li EK-M, Wang G, et al. The gene expression of type 17 T-helper cell-related cytokines in the urinary sediment of patients with systemic lupus erythematosus. Rheumatology. 2009 Dec 1;48(12):1491–7.

17. van Vollenhoven RF, Hahn BH, Tsokos GC, Wagner CL, Lipsky P, Touma Z, et al. Efficacy and safety of ustekinumab, an IL-12 and IL-23 inhibitor, in patients with active systemic lupus erythematosus: results of a multicentre, double-blind, phase 2, randomised, controlled study. Lancet Lond Engl. 2018 13;392(10155):1330–9.

18. Chasset F, Arnaud L. Targeting interferons and their pathways in systemic lupus erythematosus. Autoimmun Rev. 2018 Jan;17(1):44–52.

19. Denny MF, Yalavarthi S, Zhao W, Thacker SG, Anderson M, Sandy AR, et al. A distinct subset of proinflammatory neutrophils isolated from patients with systemic lupus erythematosus induces vascular damage and synthesizes type I IFNs. J Immunol Baltim Md 1950. 2010 Mar 15;184(6):3284–97.

20. Kaplan MJ. Neutrophils in the pathogenesis and manifestations of SLE. Nat Rev Rheumatol. 2011 Sep 27;7(12):691–9.

21. O'Gorman WE, Hsieh EWY, Savig ES, Gherardini PF, Hernandez JD, Hansmann L, et al. Single-cell systems level analysis of human toll-like-receptor activation defines a chemokine signature in systemic lupus erythematosus. J Allergy Clin Immunol. 2015 Nov;136(5):1326–36.

22. Hill GS, Delahousse M, Nochy D, Rémy P, Mignon F, Méry JP, et al. Predictive power of the second renal biopsy in lupus nephritis: significance of macrophages. Kidney Int. 2001 Jan;59(1):304–16.

23. Elkon KB, Santer DM. Complement, interferon and lupus. CurrOpin Immunol. 2012 Dec;24(6):665–70.

24. Craft JE Follicular helper T cells in immunity and systemic autoimmunity. Nat Rev Rheumatol. 2012 May 1;8 6):337–47.

25. Garrett-Sinha L, John S, Gaffen S. IL-17 and the Th17 lineage in systemic lupus erythematosus. Curr Opin Rheumatol. 2008 Sep 1;20(5):519–25.

26. Katsuyama T, Tsokos GC, Moulton VR. Aberrant T cell signaling and subsets in systemic lupus erythematosus. Front Immunol. 2018 May 17;9:1088.

27. Liphaus BL, Jesus AA, Silva CA, Coutinho A, Carneiro-Sampaio M. Increased IgE serum levels are unrelated to allergic and parasitic diseases in patients with juvenile systemic lupus erythematosus. Clinics. 2012 Nov;67(11):1275–80.
28. Dema B, Charles N, Pellefigues C, Ricks TK, Suzuki R, Jiang C, et al. Immunoglobulin E plays an immunoregulatory role in lupus. J Exp Med. 2014 Oct 20;211(11):2159–68.
29. Harvey PR, Gordon C. B-cell targeted therapies in systemic lupus erythematosus: Successes and challenges. BioDrugs Clin Immunother Biopharm Gene Ther. 2013 Apr;27(2):85–95.
30. Collison J. Low-dose IL-2 therapy for autoimmune diseases. Nat Rev Rheumatol. 2019 Jan;15(1):2.
31. Sakkas LI, Daoussis D, Mavropoulos A, Liossis SN, Bogdanos DP. Regulatory B cells: New players in inflammatory and autoimmune rheumatic diseases. Semin Arthritis Rheum. 2019 Jun;48(6):1133–1141.
32. Stannard JN, Kahlenberg JM. Cutaneous lupus erythematosus: Updates on pathogenesis and associations with systemic lupus. Curr OpinRheumatol. 2016 Sep;28(5):453–9.
33. Stock AD, Gelb S, Pasternak O, Ben-Zvi A, Putterman C. The blood brain barrier and neuropsychiatric lupus: new perspectives in light of advances in understanding the neuroimmune interface. Autoimmun Rev. 2017 Jun 1;16(6):612–9.
34. Yoshio T, Hirata D, Onda K, Nara H, Minota S. Antiribosomal P protein antibodies in cerebrospinal fluid are associated with neuropsychiatric systemic lupus erythematosus. J Rheumatol. 2005 Jan;32(1):34–9.
35. Yoshio T, Okamoto H, Hirohata S, Minota S. IgG anti-NR2 glutamate receptor autoantibodies from patients with systemic lupus erythematosus activate endothelial cells. Arthritis Rheum. 2013 Feb;65(2):457–63.
36. Steffen BJ, Breier G, Butcher EC, Schulz M, Engelhardt B. ICAM-1, VCAM-1, and MAdCAM-1 are expressed on choroid plexus epithelium but not endothelium and mediate binding of lymphocytes in vitro. Am J Pathol. 1996 Jun;148(6):1819–38.
37. Devaraju P, Gulati R, Singh BK, Mithun CB, Negi VS. The CTLA4 +49 A/G (rs231775) polymorphism influences susceptibility to SLE in South Indian Tamils. Tissue Antigens. 2014 Jun;83(6):418–21.
38. Devaraju P, Gulati R, Antony PT, Mithun CB, Negi VS. Susceptibility to SLE in South Indian Tamils may be influenced by genetic selection pressure on TLR2 and TLR9 genes. Mol Immunol. 2015 Mar 1;64(1):123–6.
39. Panneer D, Antony P, Negi V. Q222R polymorphism in DNAse I gene is a risk factor for nephritis in South Indian SLE patients. Lupus. 2013 Sep 1;22(10):996–1000.
40. Mahto H, Tripathy R, Das BK, Panda AK. Association between vitamin D receptor polymorphisms and systemic lupus erythematosus in an Indian cohort. Int J Rheum Dis. 2018 Feb;21(2):468–76.
41. Katkam SK, Rajasekhar L, Kumaraswami K, Kutala VK. Association of IL -6 -174 G>C polymorphism with the risk of SLE among south Indians: evidence from case-control study and meta-analysis. Lupus. 2017 Dec;26(14):1491–501.
42. Umare VD, Pradhan VD, Rajadhyaksha AG, Patwardhan MM, Ghosh K, Nadkarni AH. Impact of TNF-α and LTα gene polymorphisms on genetic susceptibility in Indian SLE patients. Hum Immunol. 2017 Feb;78(2):201–8.
43. Devaraju P, Reni BN, Gulati R, Mehra S, Negi VS. Complement C1q and C2 polymorphisms are not risk factors for SLE in Indian Tamils. Immunobiology. 2014 Jun;219(6):465–8.
44. Umare V, Pradhan V, Rajadhyaksha A, Ghosh K, Nadkarni A. Predisposition of IL-1β (-511 C/T) polymorphism to renal and hematologic disorders in Indian SLE patients. Gene. 2018 Jan 30;641:41–5.
45. Umare VD, Pradhan VD, Rajadhyaksha AG, Ghosh K, Nadkarni AH. A functional SNP MCP-1 (-2518A/G) predispose to renal disorder in Indian systemic lupus erythematosus patients. Cytokine. 2017;96:189–94.
46. Negi VS, Devaraju P, Misra DP, Jain VK, Usdadiya JB, Antony PT, et al. Mannose-binding lectin (MBL) codon 54 (rs1800450) polymorphism predisposes towards medium vessel vasculitis in patients with systemic lupus erythematosus. Clin Rheumatol. 2017 Apr;36(4):837–43.

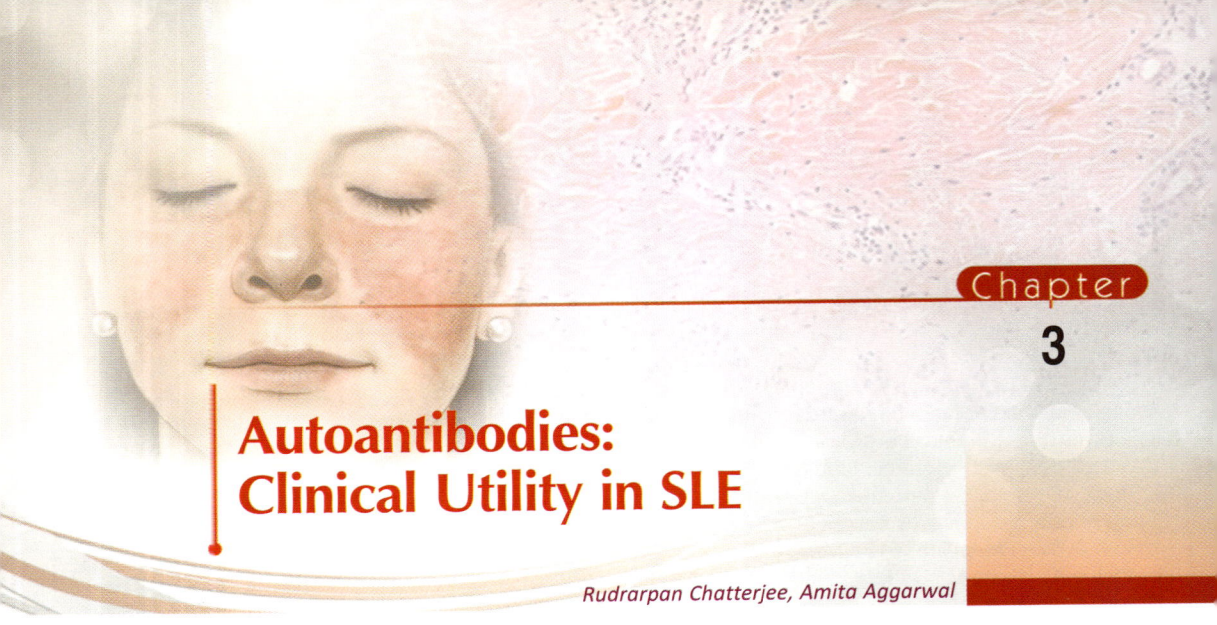

Autoantibodies: Clinical Utility in SLE

Rudrarpan Chatterjee, Amita Aggarwal

Systemic lupus erythematosus is a non-organ specific autoimmune disease characterized by an array of autoantibodies. These autoantibodies are directed against cellular components like cell membrane, cytosolic proteins, nuclear constituents, etc. Anti-nuclear antibodies (ANA) are the hall mark of SLE. These ANAs can be directed against DNA, DNA-associated proteins like histones, RNA-associated proteins like Sm, nucleolar proteins and proteins expressed during cell proliferation. The autoantibodies can help us in diagnosis and follow up of the patient.

Case 1: A 25-year-old lady has polyarthritis for 4 months and was referred as a case of rheumatoid arthritis as she was rheumatoid factor (RF) positive. Review of her routine investigations revealed that she had platelet count of 1.2 lacs and a normal CRP though her ESR was 95 mm. In view of this a possibility of lupus was thought off and her investigations later showed 4+ positive ANA, high titers of antibodies to dsDNA and low complements thus confirming a diagnosis of SLE.

As can be seen in this case that patients with SLE can have multiple autoantibodies like RF, ANA, anti-dsDNA and possibly antibodies against platelet antigens. Among these ANA is usually the first antibody to be ordered in any patient suspected to have SLE.

ANTINUCLEAR ANTIBODIES

Antinuclear antibody as the name suggest is an antibody that is against the nuclear components. It is usually detected by indirect immunofluorescence (IIF) assay.[1] This assay uses Hep2 cells which have large nuclei so that you can see the various patterns (Table 3.1). Among the various patterns homogeneous is the most specific for SLE (Fig. 3.1).

Other patterns like few nuclear dots, cytoplasmic staining is infrequently seen. The patterns can be visualized on http://www.anapatterns.org/.

Antinuclear antibodies are present in nearly 98% of patients with SLE but they are also present in many other connective tissue diseases like Sjogren syndrome, myositis, systemic sclerosis, etc. In addition, it can be seen in chronic infections, malignancies and following ingestion of certain drugs like isoniazid. Thus, because of its high sensitivity but low specificity, ANA is a good test to exclude SLE if it is negative.[2] However, a positive ANA

Table 3.1: Different patterns of anti-nuclear antibodies seen on IIF assay

Pattern	Target antigens
Homogeneous	DNA, histones, nucleosome
Speckled	
Fine	Ro (SS-A), La (SS-B)
Coarse	Sm, nRNP
Centromere	Centromeric protein A, B
Nucleolar	RNA polymerase, PM-Scl
Envelope	Laminins

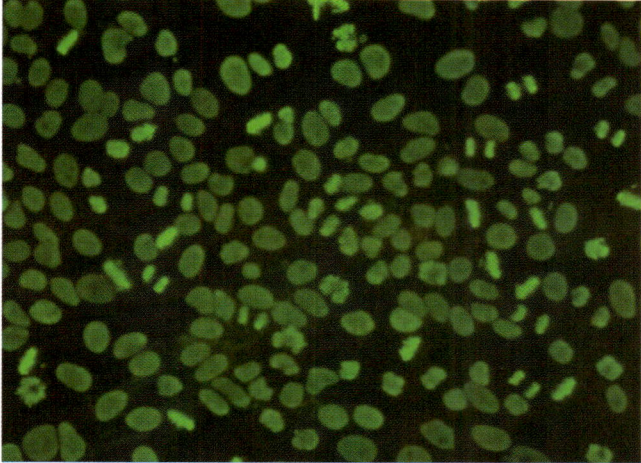

Fig. 3.1: Homogenous ANA pattern as seen on Hep2 cells using indirect immunofluorescence assay

only increases the likelihood of a diagnosis of connective tissue disease like SLE in an appropriate clinical setting.

If ANA is negative and clinical suspicion of SLE is high then anti-Ro antibodies, anti-phospholipid antibodies should be tested as they can be present in SLE patients. Further chronic renal insufficiency and use of B cell depletion therapies can also result in negative ANA in a patient with SLE.[3]

The higher the titer the more likely it is of clinical significance. Once the ANA is positive, sub-specificity testing can help in disease classification and prognostication. Presence of antibodies to dsDNA have a strong association with nephritis.

However, there is no need to repeat ANA as it stays positive throughout the life of an SLE patient and most therapies do not significantly affect its levels except B cell depletion therapy.

ANTIBODIES TO dsDNA

In the nucleus the double strand of DNA is wound around histone proteins. The antibodies can be formed against dsDNA, histones or a complex of dsDNA/histone. The complex of 100bp nucleotides along with histones are called nucleosome.[4] Antibody levels can be measured by ELISA. In addition, antibodies to dsDNA can also be detected using radio-immunoassay (Farr assay) or IIF assay using *Crithidia luciliae*.

The IIF assay is the most specific and can be used for diagnostic purpose whereas the ELISA is quantitative and thus can be used for serial monitoring of the levels of antibody.

Antibodies to dsDNA are seen in 50–60% of patients with SLE and their presence has a fair association with presence of lupus nephritis. Patients with proliferative nephritis usually have elevated anti-dsDNA antibodies. In patients who are anti-dsDNA antibody negative 10% can have anti-nucleosomal antibodies. Anti-dsDNA antibodies can contribute to SLE pathogenesis by forming immune complexes and leading to complement activation, binding to proteins on the glomerular cells and causing endothelial dysfunction, modulating gene expression of pro-inflammatory genes, etc.[5]

Antibodies to dsDNA and nucleosome correlate with disease activity and are monitored serially in the clinic along with serum C3 and C4 levels to monitor disease flares in patients. Patients with persistently elevated anti-dsDNA antibodies have higher chance of relapse, similarly in about two-thirds patients a rise in antibody level may harbinger a relapse after 3–9 months. The patients who show a rise in anti-dsDNA levels need a closer follow-up and some centers use pre-emptive increase in immunosuppression. However, most feel that the treatment should be changed when clinical relapse occurs.[6]

Extractable Nuclear Antigens

This group of antibodies derive their name from the fact that they were originally isolated by salt extraction of nuclear proteins. Currently reference laboratories use automated line immunoassays to test for these antibodies and commercial kits are available for the same. Routine commercial kits test for a panel that includes dsDNA, histones, Sm(D), nRNP, SS-A (Ro60, Ro52), SS-B(La), Ribosomal-P(P0), Jo-1, Mi-2, Topoisomerae-1 (Scl-70), PCNA, AMA-M2 and CENP-B.[7] Although Jo-1, Ribosomal P and SSA (Ro52) are cytoplasmic antigens and show a cytoplasmic staining on ANA, the term extractable nuclear antigen (ENA) has been retained to avoid confusion.

ANA tests the reactivity to the complete antigen inside the cell, whereas ENA screen consists of particular recombinant subunits which are of clinical significance (e.g. D subunit of Sm, P0 subunit of ribosomal P, B subunit of CENP). Hence, a patient who has ANA positivity may have a negative ENA screen. It is important to know when we must order an ENA screen in light of ANA positivity (Table 3.2).[8] As a general rule, a higher titre of ANA

Table 3.2: Indications for ordering ENA screen in patients who are ANA positive

ANA pattern	Indication for ENA screen
Homogenous	ENA screen for all with high titre ANA positivity. Also test for dsDNA
Speckled	ENA screen for medium and high titre ANA positivity
Atypical speckled	ENA screen for all cases irrespective of titre
	Likely to be SS-A with or without SS-B
Nucleolar	Conventional ENA screen not required
	Consider dedicated systemic sclerosis ENA panel that includes PM-Scl (75,100 kDa), fibrillarin, NOR90, Th/T0, RNA polymerase III
Centromere	ENA screen may be done to confirm CENP-B
Cytoplasmic	ENA screen for all to detect Ribosomal P(P0)
	Anti-synthetase antibodies(Jo-1, PL-7, PL-12) if clinical suspicion

positivity makes it more likely that an ENA screen will yield positive results that will help us identify possible clinical associations in a particular patient.

CLINICAL RELEVANCE IN SLE

Autoantibodies are present in patients of SLE much prior to symptomatic disease. A phase of benign autoimunity esists in which ANAs, anti-Ro, anti-La and anti-phospholipid antibodies (APLA) exist in the absence of symptomatic disease. This is followed by a phase of pathogenic autoimmunity during which the levels of circulating antibodies to dsDNA, Sm and nRNP increase and are followed by symptom onset.[9]

Antibodies exert their pathogenic effects by immune complex formation and complement activation (anti-dsDNA and nucleosome), cell surface binding and cytotoxicity (anti-Ro/La, anti-erythrocyte), cellular penetration and dysfunction (anti-dsDNA and nRNP) and binding to extracellular molecules like heparan sulphate (anti-phospholipid antibodies).[10]

Different clusters of patients with similar antibody profiles have been described. Lupus nephritis and renal damage predominates in the cluster with anti-dsDNA antibodies. Pulmonary artery hypertension and Raynaud's phenomenon are seen in the cluster with Sm/RNP antibodies. Autoimmune hemolytic anemia, thrombocytopenia, antiphospholipid syndrome and neurologic involvement predominate in the anticardiolipin and lupus anticoagulant cluster.[11] Though some studies have identified cutaneous involvement in the anti-Ro/La antibody cluster, others have found no clinical association with this.[11,12] The clinical associations of various autoantibodies may help prognosticate current and future organ involvement in patients (Table 3.3).[13]

It is also important to note that though antibodies to histone are associated with drug-induced lupus, they may be seen in most patients of SLE even without a drug trigger. Antibodies to Ro/La are an important tool in pregnancy counselling. Patients who have these antibodies are at higher risk of congenital heart block and require more stringent monitoring between 16–24 weeks of pregnancy. An ultrasound every 2–4 weeks may be prudent from 16 weeks of pregnancy in such patients. Although the risk of developing heart block is low (2%) primarily in these patients, the risk increases (12.1%) in those with a prior pregnancy with congenital heart block and these antibodies.[14,15]

Table 3.3: Clinical association of different extractable nuclear antigens in SLE		
Antigen	*Prevalence of autoantibody*	*Disease association*
dsDNA	60–90%	Nephritis, acute cutaneous lupus erythematosus.
Histones	50% (95% in drug-induced lupus)	Drug-induced lupus
Nucleosome	50–90%	Nephitis
Sm	20–40%	Nephritis, vasculitis, neurologic, hematologic
nRNP	20–30%	None
Ro60/SS-A	30–40%	Neonatal lupus, congenital heart block, subacute cutaneous lupus
Ro52/SS-A	30–40%	Neonatal lupus
La/SS-B	10–15%	Neonatal lupus, congenital heart block, subacute cutaneous lupus
Ribosomal P(P0)	10–40%	Neuropsychiatric manifestations, depression, psychosis liver disease

Prevalence in the general population

In a large study, the prevalence of ENAs in the general healthy population was found to be less than 2.5%. The presence of these antibodies did not lead to a cumulative increase in incidence of connective tissue disorders over a follow-up period of 15 years. However, ANA positivity was shown to predict lifetime risk of developing a connective tissue disease (age and sex adjusted HR 11.38, 95% CI 2.45–52.97).[16] Antibodies to SS-A (Ro52, Ro 60) are often seen in the clinic without any significant clinical symptoms. Other than the aforementioned pregnancy risk and related counselling, it is not prudent to read much into the presence of these autoantibodies.

Evolution Over Time

Although ANA levels tend to remain positive throughout life with the exception of some patients on B cell depleting therapies, the same cannot be said of ENAs. Both positive and negative seroconversion of ENAs has been seen on longitudinal follow up. Anti SS-A(Ro) and anti-nRNP antibody levels show less fluctuation compared to antibodies to dsDNA and Sm.[17] However, good agreement in the presence of antibodies to dsDNA, Sm, SS-A, SS-B and nRNP have been found over time. A positive seroconversion has been demonstrated in those with historically negative antibody status in 13% for dsDNA, 7% for Sm, 20% for nRNP, 10% for SS-A and 3% for SS-B.[18] This has practical implications in the clinic as the current ACR criteria for SLE are cumulative and historical autoantibody positivity needs to be considered when classifying a patient to enroll in a study. The persistence of these autoantibodies may also help in reinforcing the diagnosis of SLE.

ANTI-PHOSPHOLIPID ANTIBODIES

IgM, IgG and IgA antibodies to cardiolipin and β2GP-I and presence of lupus anticoagulant constitute commonly measured anti-phospholipid antibodies (APLA) (Table 3.4). 30–40% of patients of SLE have anti-phospholipid antibodies and half of them go on to develop

Table 3.4: Clinical association of antibodies other than ENAs in SLE

Antibodies related to hematological manifestations

Antiphospholipid antibodies 　Anti-cardiolipin 　Anti-β2GP-I 　Lupus anticoagulant	30–40%	Neurologic, hematologic (hemolytic anemia, thrombocytopenia), livedo reticularis, thrombotic microangiopathy, APS nephropathy.
Anti-erythrocytes antibodies 　Direct coomb's test (DCT)	10–50%	Hemolytic anemia[22]
Anti-lymphocyte antibodies	42.3%	Lymphopenia, lupus nephritis, disease activity[23]
Anti-platelet antibodies	29%	Thrombocytopenia[24]
Anti-thrombopoietin antibodies	39%	
Antibodies related to neurological manifestations		
Anti-NMDAR antibodies	30%	Depression, neuropsychiatric manifestations[25]
Anti-aquaporin 4 antibodies	Rare	Transverse myelitis, neuromyelitis optica spectrum disorders
Other antibodies		
Anti-C1q antibodies nephritis),	20–50%	Nephritis (100% of patients with proliferative lupus correlates with disease activity

APLA syndrome.[13] Anti-cardiolipin and anti β2GP-I antibodies are detected by ELISA (>40 IgM or IgG phospholipid units are taken as positive) whereas lupus anticoagulant is detected by a functional assay that measures the ability of APLA to prolong phospholipid-dependent clotting reactions such as the activated plasma thromboplastin time (aPTT), kaolin clotting time (KCT) or the dilute Russell viper venom test (DRVVT). At least two tests 12 weeks apart should be positive to label a patient to have APLA syndrome. An elevated aPTT in the absence of anticoagulation or any other anomaly may often point to a diagnosis of APLA in the clinic. Presence of antiphospholipid antibodies in SLE is associated with neurologic manifestations, thrombotic microangiopathies, APS nephropathy, worse renal outcomes and hematological abnormalities like thrombocytopenia and hemolytic anemia (Evan's syndrome) in addition to be increased risk of thrombotic events.[20-21]

ANTIBODIES RELATED TO HEMATOLOGICAL MANIFESTATIONS

The direct Coombs' test (DCT) is a simple test that is part of the criteria for classification of SLE as part of the immunological phenomenon. It is used to detect antibodies as well as complement coated antibodies on erythrocyte surfaces which is ubiquitous in SLE. A large study found evidence of autoimmune hemolysis in 54.3% of those with a positive DCT.[22] Thus, almost half of the patients with these antibodies may not have any clinical evidence of hemolysis. Anti-lymphocyte antibodies have been demonstrated to have a direct pathogenic role in lymphopenia in patients of SLE. These antibodies are also associated with presence of lupus nephritis (OR 5.87, 95% CI 2.52–13.67) and active disease (OR 3.71, 95% CI 1.56–8.83).[17] Anti-platelet antibodies may cause thrombocytopenia by direct cytolytic effects on platelets or by blocking the action of thrombopoietin.[24] However, these antibodies are not of much relevance to clinical practice as patients of SLE rarely have bleeding manifestations due to a robust bone marrow response at times of excessive platelet destruction.

ANTIBODIES RELATED TO NEUROLOGICAL MANIFESTATIONS

Antibodies to ribosomal P have been most widely reported in patients with neuropsychiatric manifestations of lupus. These antibodies have a high specificity but lack sensitivity for the diagnosis of neuropsychiatric lupus.[26, 27] The diagnostic utility of these antibodies has further been questioned by meta-analysis which found these antibodies to have a weighted sensitivity of only 26% (95% CI 15–42%) and specificity of 80% (95% CI 74–85%).[21] However, multiple studies support the association of psychosis attributed to SLE with the presence of these antibodies.[28]

Anti-NMDA glutamate receptor antibodies are a subset of anti-dsDNA antibodies that cross react with a domain of the NMDA receptor.[29] These antibodies are present in the sera, CSF as well as the brain tissue in patients of NPSLE. This suggests a breakdown in the blood brain and blood CSF barrier as a possible mechanism of action of these antibodies even in the absence of systemic inflammation. Their levels in sera and CSF are considerably elevated in patients of NPSLE and they have potential diagnostic significance.[30]

Anti-aquaporin 4 antibodies have been very rarely described in patients with NPSLE and correlate only with the presence of transverse myelitis and not with other features of NPSLE.[31]

OTHER AUTOANTIBODIES

C1q is the first component of the classical complement pathway. Antibodies to C1q have been demonstrated to activate both classic and mannose binding lectin pathway of complement activation *in vivo*.[32] By inhibiting the clearance of early apoptotic cells, these antibodies have a direct pathogenic role in patients of lupus nephritis.[33] These antibodies correlate with disease activity and the presence of lupus nephritis but are rarely used in the clinic due to non-availability of assays in routine clinical labs.

Antibodies to annexin-A2 have been recently described in kidney biopsies in patients of lupus nephritis whereas antibodies to α-actinin have been demonstrated in sera as well as kidney biopsies of patients with lupus nephritis.[13] At present these two antibodies are of academic interest alone and their relevance in clinical practice is not known.

CONCLUSION

Patients with SLE can have a wide range of autoantibodies, however in clinical practice ANA is used as a screening test followed by antibodies to dsDNA, ENA profile, APLA and DCT. Rest of the autoantibodies are used only in special situations. For follow-up only anti-dsDNA antibody is measured.

REFERENCES

1. Damoiseaux J, Andrade LEC, Carballo OG, Conrad K, Francescantonio PLC, Fritzler MJ, Garcia de la Torre I, Herold M, Klotz W, Cruvinel WM, Mimori T, vonMuhlen C, Satoh M, Chan EK. Clinical relevance of HEp-2 indirect immunofluorescent patterns: The International Consensus on ANA patterns (ICAP) perspective. Ann Rheum Dis. 2019 Jul;78(7):879–89.
2. Pisetsky DS. Anti-DNA and autoantibodies. Curr Opin Rheumatol. 2000 Sep;12(5):364–8.
3. Pisetsky DS. Evolving story of autoantibodies in systemic lupus erythematosus. J Autoimmun. 2019 Dec 3:102356.
4. Ghiggeri GM, D'Alessandro M, Bartolomeo D, Degl'Innocenti ML, Magnasco A, Lugani F, Prunotto M, Bruschi M. An update on antibodies to nucleosome components as biomarkers of systemic lupus erythematosus and of lupus flares. Int J Mol Sci. 2019 Nov 18;20(22).
5. Mummert E, Fritzler MJ, Sjöwall C, Bentow C, Mahler M. The clinical utility of anti-double-stranded DNA antibodies and the challenges of their determination. J Immunol Methods. 2018 Aug;459:11–19.
6. Floris A, Piga M, Cauli A, Mathieu A. Predictors of flares in systemic lupus erythematosus: Preventive therapeutic intervention based on serial anti-dsDNA antibodies assessment. Analysis of a monocentric cohort and literature review. Autoimmun Rev. 2016 Jul;15(7):656–63.
7. Jeong S, Hwang H, Roh J, Shim JE, Kim J, Kim GT, et al. Evaluation of an automated screening assay, compared to indirect immunofluorescence, an extractable nuclear antigen assay, and a line immunoassay in a large cohort of asian patients with antinuclear antibody-associated rheumatoid diseases: A multicenter retrospective study. J Immunol Res. 2018 May 2;2018:9094217.
8. Damoiseaux JGMC, Cohen Tervaert JW. From ANA to ENA: How to proceed? Autoimmun Rev. 2006 Jan;5(1):10–7.
9. Arbuckle MR, McClain MT, Rubertone MV, Scofield RH, Dennis GJ, James JA, et al. Development of autoantibodies before the clinical onset of systemic lupus erythematosus. N Engl J Med. 2003 Oct 16; 349(16):1526–33.
10. Gualtierotti R, Biggioggero M, Penatti AE, Meroni PL. Updating on the pathogenesis of systemic lupus erythematosus. Autoimmun Rev. 2010 Nov;10(1):3–7.
11. Artim-Esen B, Çene E, Sahinkaya Y, Ertan S, Pehlivan Ö, Kamali S, et al. Cluster analysis of autoantibodies in 852 patients with systemic lupus erythematosus from a single center. J Rheumatol. 2014 Jul;41(7):1304–10.
12. Tang X, Huang Y, Deng W, Tang L, Weng W, Zhang X. Clinical and serologic correlations and autoantibody clusters in systemic lupus erythematosus: a retrospective review of 917 patients in South China. Medicine (Baltimore). 2010 Jan;89(1):62–7.
13. Dema B, Charles N. Autoantibodies in SLE: Specificities, isotypes and receptors. Antibodies Basel Switz. 2016 Jan 4;5(1).

14. Brucato A, Frassi M, Franceschini F, Cimaz R, Faden D, Pisoni MP, et al. Risk of congenital complete heart block in newborns of mothers with anti-Ro/SSA antibodies detected by counter-immunoelectrophoresis: a prospective study of 100 women. Arthritis Rheum. 2001 Aug;44(8):1832–5.

15. Ambrosi A, Salomonsson S, Eliasson H, Zeffer E, Skog A, Dzikaite V, et al. Development of heart block in children of SSA/SSB-autoantibody-positive women is associated with maternal age and displays a season-of-birth pattern. Ann Rheum Dis. 2012 Mar;71(3):334–40.

16. Selmi C, Ceribelli A, Generali E, Scirè CA, Alborghetti F, Colloredo G, et al. Serum antinuclear and extractable nuclear antigen antibody prevalence and associated morbidity and mortality in the general population over 15years. Autoimmun Rev. 2016 Feb;15(2):162–6.

17. Faria AC, Barcellos KSA, Andrade LEC. Longitudinal fluctuation of antibodies to extractable nuclear antigens in systemic lupus erythematosus. J Rheumatol. 2005 Jul;32(7):1267–72.

18. Ippolito A, Wallace DJ, Gladman D, Fortin PR, Urowitz M, Werth V, et al. Autoantibodies in systemic lupus erythematosus: comparison of historical and current assessment of seropositivity. Lupus. 2011 Mar;20(3):250–5.

19. Sciascia S, Cuadrado MJ, Khamashta M, Roccatello D. Renal involvement in antiphospholipid syndrome. Nat Rev Nephrol. 2014 May;10(5):279–89.

20. Cervera R, Piette J-C, Font J, Khamashta MA, Shoenfeld Y, Camps MT, et al. Antiphospholipid syndrome: clinical and immunologic manifestations and patterns of disease expression in a cohort of 1,000 patients. Arthritis Rheum. 2002 Apr;46(4):1019–27.

21. Stojanovich L, Djokovic A, Stanisavljevic N, Zdravkovic M. The cutaneous manifestations are significantly related to cerebrovascular in a Serbian cohort of patients with Hughes syndrome. Lupus. 2018 Apr;27(5):858–63.

22. Skare T, Picelli L, Dos Santos TAG, Nisihara R. Direct antiglobulin (Coombs) test in systemic lupus erythematosus patients. Clin Rheumatol. 2017 Sep;36(9):2141–4.

23. Li C, Mu R, Lu X, He J, Jia R, Li Z. Antilymphocyte antibodies in systemic lupus erythematosus: Association with disease activity and lymphopenia. J Immunol Res [Internet]. 2014 [cited 2020 Apr 4];2014. Available from: https://www.ncbi.nlm.nih.gov/pmc/articles/PMC4016860/

24. Ziakas PD, Routsias JG, Giannouli S, Tasidou A, Tzioufas AG, Voulgarelis M. Suspects in the tale of lupus-associated thrombocytopenia. Clin Exp Immunol. 2006 Jul;145(1):71–80.

25. Husebye ES. Autoantibodies to a NR2A peptide of the glutamate/NMDA receptor in sera of patients with systemic lupus erythematosus. Ann Rheum Dis. 2005 Aug 1;64(8):1210–3.

26. Mahler M, Kessenbrock K, Szmyrka M, Takasaki Y, Garcia-De La Torre I, Shoenfeld Y, et al. International multicenter evaluation of autoantibodies to ribosomal P proteins. Clin Vaccine Immunol. 2006 Jan;13(1):77–83.

27. Karassa FB, Afeltra A, Ambrozic A, Chang D-M, De Keyser F, Doria A, et al. Accuracy of anti-ribosomal P protein antibody testing for the diagnosis of neuropsychiatric systemic lupus erythematosus: An international meta-analysis. Arthritis Rheum. 2006 Jan;54(1):312–24.

28. Sciascia S, Bertolaccini ML, Roccatello D, Khamashta MA, Sanna G. Autoantibodies involved in neuropsychiatric manifestations associated with systemic lupus erythematosus: a systematic review. J Neurol. 2014 Sep;261(9):1706–14.

29. DeGiorgio LA, Konstantinov KN, Lee SC, Hardin JA, Volpe BT, Diamond B. A subset of lupus anti-DNA antibodies cross-reacts with the NR2 glutamate receptor in systemic lupus erythematosus. Nat Med. 2001 Nov;7(11):1189–93.

30. Su D, Liu R, Li X, Sun L. Possible novel biomarkers of organ involvement in systemic lupus erythematosus. Clin Rheumatol. 2014 Aug;33(8):1025–31.

31. Závada J, Nytrová P, Wandinger KP, Jarius S, Svobodová R, Probst C, et al. Seroprevalence and specificity of NMO-IgG (anti-aquaporin 4 antibodies) in patients with neuropsychiatric systemic lupus erythematosus. Rheumatol Int. 2013 Jan;33(1):259–63.

32. Thanei S, Vanhecke D, Trendelenburg M. Anti-C1q autoantibodies from systemic lupus erythematosus patients activate the complement system via both the classical and lectin pathways. Clin Immunol Orlando Fla. 2015 Oct;160(2):180–7.

33. Pang Y, Yang X-W, Song Y, Yu F, Zhao M-H. Anti-C1q autoantibodies from active lupus nephritis patients could inhibit the clearance of apoptotic cells and complement classical pathway activation mediated by C1q in vitro. Immunobiology. 2014 Dec;219(12):980–9.

Aches and Pains in SLE

Naman Jain, Yogesh Mann Singh

INTRODUCTION

Aches and pains are one of the most common manifestations in SLE. They have been described in 53 to 95% of patients and in majority these symptoms are present at presentation.[1-5] Musculoskeletal (MSK) involvement can have a significant impact on quality of life and is associated with work disability.[6,7] Active disease affecting the MSK system is frequent and constitutes 58% of disease flares.[1] Damage accrual in the MSK system was found about 24% of Hopkins lupus cohort.[1] MSK damage is a poor prognostic marker and is associated with increased mortality rates.[8] MSK manifestations can affect joint, muscle, bone and supporting structures. These include arthritis and arthralgia, tenosynovitis, myositis, osteoporosis, fibromyalgia and osteonecrosis. In addition, infection of MSK systems can occur in SLE due to immunosuppressive drugs.[5]

Case 1: A 25-year-female presented with 1 year history of intermittent symmetrical joint pain and swelling associated with morning stiffness involving both hands, wrist, shoulder and knee joints. She required help for activities of daily living. She also had complaints of fever, oral ulcer and fatigue. However, she denied history of Raynaud's phenomenon or sicca symptoms.

On examination she had active polyarthritis and palatal ulcer. Labs revealed anemia and elevated ESR of 56 mm and CRP of 2.36 mg/dl. Urine analysis, liver function and renal function tests were normal. Direct Coombs' test and ANA was positive. In addition, she had rheumatoid factor, anti-dsDNA, anti-nucleosome and anti-ribosomal antibodies. Complement were low. Rheumatoid factor (RF) was positive. Anti-cyclic citrullinated peptide antibody (Anti-CCP) was negative. She was treated with steroids, hydroxychloroquine sulfate (HCQs) and azathioprine (AZA) with which she had good response.

Though this patient has polyarthritis and RF was positive, the patient was diagnosed to have SLE as she had extra-articular features (fever, oral ulcers) and lab results (ANA, ENA screen, complement levels) supporting the diagnosis of SLE. Thus, every patient with polyarthritis need to have a detailed system review as well as review of investigations.

JOINT MANIFESTATIONS

Joint involvement at presentation is common in SLE and can occur in 60 to 95% of patients during the disease course.[5] In 30 to 50% of patients with SLE, articular involvement is the initial symptom.[1,2] They can precede the diagnosis of SLE by months to years and are associated with increased risk of work loss and workplace impairment.[2,9,10] The symptoms of articular involvement may include joint pain, swelling and stiffness. Morning stiffness is a frequent complaint but it usually lasts for a few minutes and is not as prolonged as in RA. In about 33% of patients, morning stiffness may be absent.[2]

Arthralgias are the most common manifestation of lupus joint involvement both at the onset and during the course of the disease.[1] Pain due to arthralgia is often extremely intense and disproportionate to the finding at the physical examination. Tumulty, et al. initially described this paradox in 1954 as characteristic of lupus joint involvement. In the Hopkins lupus cohort, arthralgia and arthritis were observed in 90 and 80% of patients with SLE, respectively.[1] Another feature described as characteristic of lupus arthritis is marked soft tissue swelling which is often present in the hands. Unlike rheumatoid arthritis (RA), the swelling may not be localized to joints alone. The swelling is diffusely present over the entire dorsum of wrist, hands and fingers.[4] Arthritis in SLE can be polyarticular or oligoarticular. Mono-articular involvement is rare.[2] The typical pattern is symmetrical, similar to that seen in rheumatoid arthritis. However, asymmetric patterns can also be seen.[2] All major and minor joints may be affected. Commonly affected joints include the wrists, knees, ankles, elbows and shoulders, in that order of prevalence. Arthritis in the course of the disease can be migratory, episodic or persistent.[2] Chronic or persistent arthritis as defined as persistent arthritis for at least 6 weeks is rare and seen in <5% of patients with SLE.[11] There is variability with regards to the severity of arthritis ranging from arthralgia or mild arthritis to severe erosive and/or deforming arthritis with functional disability.

Traditionally, three types of arthritis have been described in SLE: Non-deforming and non-erosive arthritis, Jaccoud's arthropathy and Rhupus.

A. Non-deforming and Non-erosive Arthritis

This is the most common form of arthritis seen in SLE. This description was based on absence of deformities on clinical examination and absence of erosions on conventional radiology. However, recent studies using either high-resolution ultrasonography (HRUS) or magnetic resonance imaging (MRI) have shown the presence of erosions in this subset of lupus patients.[6]

B. Jaccoud's Arthropathy

Jaccoud's arthropathy (JA) is a deforming, non-erosive arthropathy which was initially described in association with rheumatic fever but has been seen in other rheumatological disorders including SLE. Its prevalence in SLE is about 3–5%.[12,13] It mainly affects the hands, but has been described in the feet, knee and shoulder.[13-15] Deformities affecting the hand include ulnar deviation, swan neck, 'z'-thumb and 'boutonniere' (Fig. 4.1a and 1b). Deformities of the feet ('lupus feet') include hallux valgus, hammer toes and/or subluxation of the metatarsophalangeal joint.[15] These deformities result from joint capsule laxity with subsequent fibrosis, muscle atrophy, and tendon contracture.

A classical radiographic feature of JA is the hook lesion observed on the palmar-radial surface of the metacarpal heads seen in plain radiograph of the hands.[14] However, these lesions are not pathognomonic for JA and can be seen in conditions like RA, gout, pseudo-gout and osteoarthritis.Though X-rays donot show erosions, HRUS and MRI have shown erosive changes in JA.[14]

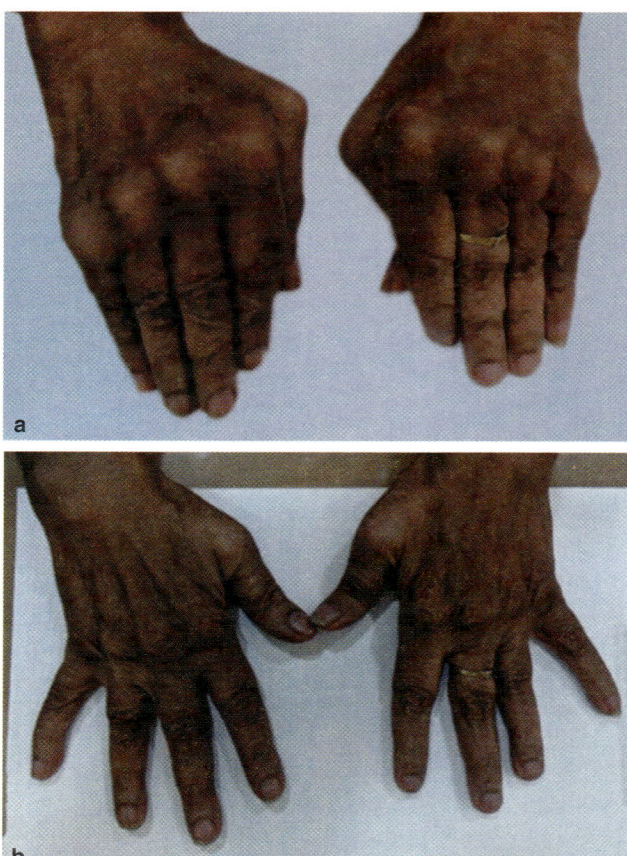

Fig. 4.1a and b: Jaccoud's arthropathy: Reversible deformity affecting the hands

C. Rhupus

Rhupus is an erosive arthritis seen in SLE. In 1971, Peter Schur coined the term 'Rhupus' to describe SLE patients with arthritis who also fulfill the classification criteria for RA. It is rare and seen in <5% of SLE patients.[12]

Rheumatoid Factor and Anti-CCP Antibodies

Rheumatoid factor (RF) though seen more often in rheumatoid arthritis (RA) can be seen in 40–50% of patients with SLE. In SLE, presence of RF is not associated with joint involvement, but with Sicca syndrome and a lower prevalence of nephropathy.[16]

Anti-CCP antibody, a more specific antibody for RA is reported in 4.4–27.3% of patients with SLE. However in SLE patients with arthritis, anti-CCP antibodies may be present in up to 50% of patients and is associated with erosive arthritis.[16,17]

Treatment

In the absence of clinical trials for treatment of lupus arthritis, the treatment is based on lines of RA and case series of lupus arthritis. The treatment includes hydroxychloroquine sulfate (HCQs) as a background agent. The dose of oral glucocorticoids (GCs) is usually dictated by underlying lupus activity. Intra-articular GCs may be indicated especially when arthritis is limited to one or few joints or in tenosynovitis. Disease modifying anti-rheumatic drugs (DMARDs) and immunosuppressive agents (IS) can be used in lupus arthritis, which is refractory to HCQs and background glucocorticoids. Methotrexate is a reasonable option in these cases. Other agents like leflunomide (LEF), azathioprine (AZA) and cyclosporine (CSA) can be considered in cases refractory to MTX.[18]

Biologics can be considered in lupus arthritis which is refractory to DMARDs/IS agents. Rituximab (RTX) has shown efficacy in RA. There are no trials in lupus arthritis. There are some reports, which have shown efficacy of RTX in lupus arthritis.[19] Though anti-TNF agents have been shown to induce autoantibodies and lupus-like syndromes, case series have shown that treatment with anti-TNF agents is beneficial in lupus arthritis. Belimumab is a newly approved biologic agent for SLE, having demonstrated benefit across organ systems including the musculoskeletal system. Other biologic agents, such as abatacept and tocilizumab have shown benefit in case series.[20,21] There is a need for further evaluation of the role of biologic agents in treatment of lupus arthritis.

TENDON INVOLVEMENT

There is a lack of clinical description of tenosynovitis in most of the lupus series. Studies using HRUS have shown that tenosynovitis occurs in 28–65% of the SLE patients.[12,22] The extensor and flexor tendons of the wrists are mainly affected.

Tendon rupture has been well documented.[23] The risk factors for tendon rupture include trauma, male gender, long-term oral steroid administration, intra-articular injections, Jaccoud's arthritis, and/or long disease duration.[23] Almost all occur in weight-bearing areas, especially in tendons about the knee (65%; most are infra-patellar) and ankle (Achilles tendon; 27%).

Subcutaneous nodules near tendons can be found in SLE in 3–13% of patients.[4,5,28] They are mainly found on the flexor tendons of the hand. Histologically, the appearance is similar to rheumatoid nodules.[23]

Case 2: A 24-year-old female presented with intermittent fever; photosensitive malar rash; polyarthritis and Raynaud's phenomenon. In addition, she had progressive difficulty in stepping up and down the staircase, standing from sitting position, combing hair and cleaning shelves. On examination she had an erythematous malar rash but no Heliotrope rash or gottron's papules, active synovitis of small joints of hand and proximal muscle weakness (Grade IV/V). Lab results showed Coomb's positive hemolytic anemia, ANA positivity, low complement levels, and elevated CPK of 1140 IU/l, ESR of 55 mm/hr and CRP of 2.3 mg/dl. Urine analysis was normal. ENA screen showed antibodies to Smith, nRNP, Ro and nucleosomes. A diagnosis of SLE with inflammatory myositis was made and she was treated with prednisolone 1 mg/kg along with HCQs and azathioprine.

MUSCLE INVOLVEMENT

Muscle involvement can occur in the form of myalgias and weakness and is seen in up to 40 to 80% of patients with SLE. Myalgias can occur during disease exacerbations and may reflect overall disease activity. Muscle involvement in SLE is usually mild and it is usually present at onset along with other systemic manifestations. Treatment of myalgias is symptomatic and is dictated by overall lupus disease activity levels and exclusion of other causes like drugs and infections.

Inflammatory myopathy is rare and seen in about 5–10% of lupus patients. It is similar to idiopathic inflammatory myopathy (IIM) in terms of clinical presentation, elevation of muscle enzymes and muscle biopsy findings as well as severity.[24] Most of the patients have a relapsing and remitting course. In clinical practice, muscle biopsy is not needed and may be done in refractory cases or when other causes, such as drugs, need to be excluded. Muscle biopsy shows evidence of myositis like inflammatory infiltrate in perivascular, perimysial distribution and in some cases extending to endomysium.[25]

Lupus with myositis can be differentiated from dermatomyositis based on characteristics of skin rash.[26,27] Lupus rash spares the nasolabial folds, whereas the rash of dermatomyositis involves the nasolabial folds. Examination of the hands can provide additional clues-Lupus rash involves the inter-joint spaces and spares the joints; dermatomyositis rash involves the joints and spares the inter-joint spaces (Gottron's papules).The scalp involvement in dermatomyositis tends to have diffuse scalp involvement and is pruritic.[26] Heliotrope rash, shawl sign, V sign and poikiloderma are characteristics of dermatomyositis.Lower extremity involvement is more commonly seen with dermatomyositis.[26]

Treatment of myositis is similar to IIM. It may include high dose GCs (including high dose pulse therapy) and use of immunosuppressive agents (methotrexate, azathioprine, MMF).[18] Intravenous cyclophosphamide and biologics may be considered in refractory myositis.[18]

In lupus patients with muscle weakness other conditions like drug-induced myopathy (e.g. GCs, antimalarials, statins), endocrinopathies, and neuropathies also need to be considered.

Drug-induced myopathy is usually reversible upon discontinuation of the offending drug (statins, antimalarials).

Case 3: A 32-year-old female was diagnosed as SLE with lupus nephritis and treated with pulse methylprednisolone (1 g/day × 3 days) followed by oral glucocorticoids. In addition, Mycophenolate mofetil (MMF) and HCQs were also started. Steroids were gradually tapered to 5 mg/day.

Two years later she developed autoimmune hemolytic anemia which required pulses of methylprednisolone (1 g/day × 3 days) followed by prednisolone 1 mg/kg tapering 5 mg every week. In between she has mild flares of arthritis and skin disease requiring escalation of glucocorticoid dosages. Following a trivial fall, she presented with acute-onset localized low back pain without motor, sensory, or bladder bowel involvement. X-ray showed osteoporosis with multiple vertebral fracture. DEXA scan revealed lumbar spine T score of 3.8. Her complete hemogram, ESR, CRP, renal function, liver function, serum calcium, phosphorus, PTH and vitamin D3 level were normal. Serum protein electrophoresis did not show any evidence of monoclonal gammopathy. She was started on teriparatide 20 mcg subcutaneously once daily.

OSTEOPOROSIS

Osteoporosis is characterized by reduced bone mass and micro-architecture deterioration of bone tissue that leads to an increased risk for bone fragility and fracture.[28] In SLE, osteoporotic fracture and resultant damage accrual forms a major part of musculoskeletal damage.[15] Approximately, 40% of patients with musculoskeletal damage have osteoporotic fractures.[3] The prevalence of osteoporosis ranges from 4.0 to 48.8%. In women with SLE, fracture risk is nearly 5-fold compared with healthy women of a similar age.[29] Symptomatic osteoporotic fractures occur in 6–12.5% of patients.[29] Frequent sites for fractures are the hip/femur, vertebra, rib, foot, ankle, and arm.

In SLE, apart from the traditional risk factors, GC use is well known risk factor. Higher daily dose as well as cumulative dose are associated with increased risk of fracture.[30] Other risk factors include chronic inflammation and active disease (low C4); serological factors (anti-Sm, anti-Ro); low androgenic state; ovarian failure; concomitant thyroid disease; metabolic factors (low vitamin D, hyper-homocystinemia); renal dysfunction and ovarian failure.[29]

Prevention and Treatment

Recent guidelines are available from various societies on how to manage these patients.[28-31] Briefly, important elements in management include lifestyle modification like avoiding smoking, limiting alcohol intake, maintaining a normal body weight, preventing falls, and performing regular weight-bearing exercise.

GCs should be used in the lowest possible dose for the shortest period of time. Administration of calcium and vitamin D in adequate doses is must. Pharmacological agents used in treatment of osteoporosis include bisphosphonates, teriparatide and denosumab.

Case 4: A 28-year-old female was diagnosed with SLE and was started on low dose prednisolone, HCQs for symptoms of polyarthritis, rash and fever. During routine review, she complained of diffuse aches and pains, polyarthralgia, non-refreshing sleep. The pain increased on activities and was better at rest. She didn't have any early morning stiffness. On clinical examination there were no features of active arthritis. She had multiple tender points. All lab investigations including inflammatory markers (ESR—16 mm, CRP—1.9 mg/L) were normal. She was diagnosed as fibromyalgia-associated with SLE.

FIBROMYALGIA

All pains in SLE are not due to active arthritis or active SLE. In patients presenting with non-specific aches/pain, absence of active arthritis, presence of tender points in an otherwise well controlled disease activity it should raise a suspicion of fibromyalgia.

Fibromyalgia (FM) is a disorder characterized by chronic, widespread musculoskeletal pain. The prevalence rates of fibromyalgia in patients with SLE range from 5 to 25%.[2,32-35] Fibromyalgia has an adverse impact on quality of life and is associated with significant disability.[36,37] Therefore, it is important that in patients with SLE, FM is identified and treated appropriately to minimize its effects on quality of life.

Treatment of FM requires both a pharmacological and a non-pharmacological approach. The non-pharmacological measures include patient education and self-management, exercises and cognitive behavioral therapy. The drugs include anti-depressants, particularly those with mixed reuptake inhibitors of serotonin and norepinephrine, such as duloxetine and milnacipran, and other agents useful for neuropathic pain, such as gabapentin and pregabalin.

Case 5: A 27-year-old female had a long history of SLE of 4 years with class III lupus nephritis at onset requiring pulse methylprednisolone and prednisolone along with MMF and HCQs. After 4 years while she was on maintenance treatment with prednisolone 5 mg per day. MMF 2 g/day and HCQs 200 mg/day she had a relapse with macrophage activation syndrome which again required high dose dexamethasone.
Now she presented with 2 months history of dull aching persistent pain over both groin which increased on walking or climbing stairs and was relieved on resting. On examination movement of both hip joints were restricted. Xray of the pelvis was normal, while MRI showed osteonecrosis of both hip joints (Stage 2 Ficat and Arlet classification). She was referred to orthopedic surgeons and underwent core decompression of the both hip joints.

OSTEONECROSIS

Osteonecrosis (ON) is also known as aseptic vascular necrosis, or ischemic necrosis of bone. ON is caused by death of bone marrow and trabecular bone due to compromised arterial blood supply.[38] In patients with SLE undergoing joint replacement ON is the major underlying cause.[39] The prevalence of ON in SLE varies from 2.1–44%.[40] Hip joints are the most commonly affected (Fig. 4.2). However, other joint areas including the knees, shoulders, wrists and ankles can also be affected. In SLE ON can also be multifocal.[41,42]

In patients with SLE, glucocorticoid (GC) use has been consistently identified as a risk. Important risk factors with GCs use include cumulative dose, peak daily dose, mean daily dose, duration of use of high doses and use of methylprednisolone pulses.[38,40] The time interval between steroid use and the development of ON varies ranging from 1 to 16 months. When compared to other diseases, the incidence of GCs related ON is much higher in SLE suggesting other factors intrinsic to SLE may be contributing this increased risk.[43] These risk factors include vasculitis, Raynaud's phenomenon, cytotoxic treatment, high disease activity, production of inflammatory mediators, defects in fibrinolysis, gene polymorphisms, antiphospholipid syndrome/antibody, and other hypercoagulable states.[38,40]

ON should be suspected in any patient with SLE who presents with persistent joint pains, especially if GCs have been used as treatment. The onset of pain is insidious and aggravated by weight bearing and ambulation. Imaging studies are required to confirm the diagnosis. In early stages, plain radiographs can be normal. MRI is the imaging modality of choice especially in early disease.[37]

Early diagnosis is crucial to the successful treatment of ON. Non-surgical treatment of osteonecrosis includes avoiding weight bearing on the affected joint, use of analgesic medications, and physiotherapy. These measures are effective only in the early stages. They provide symptomatic relief and do not seem to alter the natural course of the disease.

Surgical management of ON includes joint preserving procedures (core decompression, structural bone grafting, vascularized fibula grafting), osteotomy, resurfacing arthroplasty, hemiarthroplasty, and total joint replacement. The timing and type of surgical intervention depends on the involved site and the stage of ON. In the pre-collapse stage, the contour of the joint surfaces is maintained and joint-preserving procedures are indicated for these types of lesions.[40] The rationale of joint-preserving procedures is to reduce intraosseous

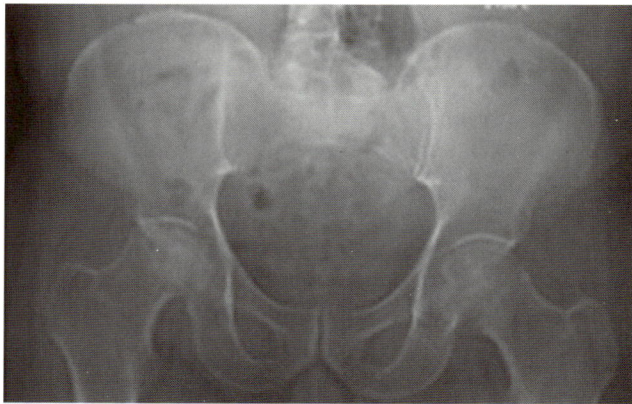

Fig. 4.2: AVN hip: Radiograph showing AVN affecting the right hip joint

pressure and intramedullary pressure; increase blood flow to the necrotic subchondral bone; and provide structural support to overlying subchondral bone. For post-collapse lesions joint-preserving procedures are not indicated due to high failure rates. In such cases, joint arthroplasty and other surgical procedures are indicated.[40]

CONCLUSION

MSK involvement in SLE is common. The involvement ranges from active disease (arthralgia/arthritis, myalgia/myositis) to conditions associated with damage (joint deformities, muscle atrophy, osteoporosis, and osteonecrosis) as a consequence of long-term disease or as a complication of treatment (GCs). MSK involvement is associated with significant morbidity, has adverse impact on quality of life and increases the risk of work loss and workplace impairment. Early recognition and adequate control of lupus disease activity are essential in prevention of the long-term sequelae associated with these conditions. GCs are associated with damage accrual in the MSK system. There is a need for treatment regimens wherein exposure to GCs can be avoided or minimized. Fibromyalgia has an adverse impact on quality of life. Therefore, it is important that in patients with SLE, FM is identified and treated appropriately to minimize its effects on quality of life.

REFERENCES

1. Petri M. Musculoskeletal complications of systemic lupus erythematosus in the Hopkins Lupus Cohort: an update. Arthritis Care Res Off J Arthritis Health Prof Assoc. 1995 Sep;8(3):137–45.
2. Labowitz R, Schumacher HR. Articular manifestations of systemic lupus erythematosus. Ann Intern Med. 1971 Jun;74(6):911–21.
3. Pistiner M, Wallace DJ, Nessim S, Metzger AL, Klinenberg JR. Lupus erythematosus in the 1980s: a survey of 570 patients. Semin Arthritis Rheum. 1991 Aug;21(1):55–64.
4. Dubois EL, Tuffanelli DL. Clinical manifestations of systemic lupus erythematosus: computer analysis of 520 cases. JAMA. 1964 Oct 12;190(2):104–11.
5. Cervera R, Khamashta MA, Font J, Sebastiani GD, Gil A, Lavilla P, et al. Systemic lupus erythematosus: clinical and immunologic patterns of disease expression in a cohort of 1,000 patients. The European Working Party on Systemic Lupus Erythematosus. Medicine (Baltimore). 1993 Mar;72(2):113–24.
6. Mahmoud K, Zayat A, Vital EM. Musculoskeletal manifestations of systemic lupus erythmatosus. Curr Opin Rheumatol. 2017 Sep;29(5):486–92.
7. Piga M, Congia M, Gabba A, Figus F, Floris A, Mathieu A, et al. Musculoskeletal manifestations as determinants of quality of life impairment in patients with systemic lupus erythematosus. Lupus. 2018 Feb;27(2):190–8.
8. Pego-Reigosa JM, Lois-Iglesias A, Rúa-Figueroa Í, Galindo M, Calvo-Alén J, de Uña-Álvarez J, et al. Relationship between damage clustering and mortality in systemic lupus erythematosus in early and late stages of the disease: Cluster analyses in a large cohort from the Spanish Society of Rheumatology Lupus Registry. Rheumatol Oxf Engl. 2016;55(7):1243–50.
9. Yelin E, Tonner C, Trupin L, Gansky SA, Julian L, Katz P, et al. Longitudinal study of the impact of incident organ manifestations and increased disease activity on work loss among persons with systemic lupus erythematosus. Arthritis Care Res. 2012 Feb;64(2):169–75.
10. Drenkard C, Bao G, Dennis G, Kan HJ, Jhingran PM, Molta CT, et al. Burden of systemic lupus erythematosus on employment and work productivity: Data from a large cohort in the southeastern United States. Arthritis Care Res. 2014 Jun;66(6):878–87.
11. Gormezano NWS, Silva CA, Aikawa NE, Barros DL, da Silva MA, Otsuzi CI, et al. Chronic arthritis in systemic lupus erythematosus: distinct features in 336 paediatric and 1830 adult patients. Clin Rheumatol. 2016 Jan;35(1):227–31.

12. Ball EMA, Bell AL. Lupus arthritis—do we have a clinically useful classification? Rheumatol Oxf Engl. 2012 May;51(5):771–9.
13. Santiago MB, Galvão V. Jaccoud arthropathy in systemic lupus erythematosus: analysis of clinical characteristics and review of the literature. Medicine (Baltimore). 2008 Jan;87(1):37–44.
14. Santiago MB. Miscellaneous non-inflammatory musculoskeletal conditions. Jaccoud's arthropathy. Best Pract Res Clin Rheumatol. 2011 Oct;25(5):715–25.
15. Saketkoo LA, Quinet R. Revisiting Jaccoud arthropathy as an ultrasound diagnosed erosive arthropathy in systemic lupus erythematosus. J Clin Rheumatol Pract Rep Rheum Musculoskelet Dis. 2007 Dec;13(6):322–7.
16. Ceccarelli F, Perricone C, Cipriano E, Massaro L, Natalucci F, Capalbo G, et al. Joint involvement in systemic lupus erythematosus: From pathogenesis to clinical assessment. Semin Arthritis Rheum. 2017;47(1):53–64.
17. Budhram A, Chu R, Rusta-Sallehy S, Ioannidis G, Denburg JA, Adachi JD, et al. Anti-cyclic citrullinated peptide antibody as a marker of erosive arthritis in patients with systemic lupus erythematosus: a systematic review and meta-analysis. Lupus. 2014 Oct;23(11):1156–63.
18. Jordan N, D'Cruz D. Current and emerging treatment options in the management of lupus. ImmunoTargets Ther. 2016;5:9–20.
19. Gracia-Tello B, Ezeonyeji A, Isenberg D. The use of rituximab in newly diagnosed patients with systemic lupus erythematosus: long-term steroid saving capacity and clinical effectiveness. Lupus Sci Med. 2017;4(1):e000182.
20. Danion F, Rosine N, Belkhir R, Gottenberg JE, Hachulla E, Chatelus E, et al. Efficacy of abatacept in systemic lupus erythematosus: a retrospective analysis of 11 patients with refractory disease. Lupus. 2016 Nov;25(13):1440–7.
21. Illei GG, Shirota Y, Yarboro CH, Daruwalla J, Tackey E, Takada K, et al. Tocilizumab in systemic lupus erythematosus: data on safety, preliminary efficacy, and impact on circulating plasma cells from an open-label phase I dosage-escalation study. Arthritis Rheum. 2010 Feb;62(2):542–52.
22. Zayat AS, Md Yusof MY, Wakefield RJ, Conaghan PG, Emery P, Vital EM. The role of ultrasound in assessing musculoskeletal symptoms of systemic lupus erythematosus: a systematic literature review. Rheumatol Oxf Engl. 2016 Mar;55(3):485–94.
23. Zoma A. Musculoskeletal involvement in systemic lupus erythematosus. Lupus. 2004;13(11):851–3.
24. Garton MJ, Isenberg DA. Clinical features of lupus myositis versus idiopathic myositis: a review of 30 cases. Br J Rheumatol. 1997 Oct;36(10):1067–74.
25. Jakati S, Rajasekhar L, Uppin M, Challa S. SLE myopathy: a clinicopathological study. Int J Rheum Dis. 2015 Nov;18(8):886–91.
26. Callen JP. Cutaneous manifestations of dermatomyositis and their management. Curr Rheumatol Rep. 2010 Jun;12(3):192–7.
27. Gilliam JN, Sontheimer RD. Distinctive cutaneous subsets in the spectrum of lupus erythematosus. J Am Acad Dermatol. 1981 Apr;4(4):471–5.
28. Qaseem A, Forciea MA, McLean RM, Denberg TD, Clinical Guidelines Committee of the American College of Physicians. Treatment of low bone density or osteoporosis to prevent fractures in men and women: A Clinical Practice Guideline Update From the American College of Physicians. Ann Intern Med. 2017 Jun 6;166(11):818–39.
29. Bultink IEM. Osteoporosis and fractures in systemic lupus erythematosus. Arthritis Care Res. 2012 Jan;64(1):2–8.
30. Buckley L, Guyatt G, Fink HA, Cannon M, Grossman J, Hansen KE, et al. 2017 American College of Rheumatology Guideline for the Prevention and Treatment of Glucocorticoid-Induced Osteoporosis. Arthritis Care Res. 2017;69(8):1095–110.
31. Cosman F, de Beur SJ, LeBoff MS, Lewiecki EM, Tanner B, Randall S, et al. Clinician's Guide to Prevention and Treatment of Osteoporosis. Osteoporos Int. 2014;25(10):2359–81.
32. Wolfe F, Petri M, Alarcón GS, Goldman J, Chakravarty EF, Katz RS, et al. Fibromyalgia, systemic lupus erythematosus (SLE), and evaluation of SLE activity. J Rheumatol. 2009 Jan;36(1):82–8.
33. Middleton GD, McFarlin JE, Lipsky PE. The prevalence and clinical impact of fibromyalgia in systemic lupus erythematosus. Arthritis Rheum. 1994 Aug;37(8):1181–8.

34. Handa R, Aggarwal P, Wali JP, Wig N, Dwivedi SN. Fibromyalgia in Indian patients with SLE. Lupus. 1998;7(7):475–8.
35. Friedman AW, Tewi MB, Ahn C, McGwin G, Fessler BJ, Bastian HM, et al. Systemic lupus erythematosus in three ethnic groups: XV. Prevalence and correlates of fibromyalgia. Lupus. 2003;12(4):274–9.
36. Kuriya B, Gladman DD, Ibañez D, Urowitz MB. Quality of life over time in patients with systemic lupus erythematosus. Arthritis Rheum. 2008 Feb 15;59(2):181–5.
37. Kiani AN, Strand V, Fang H, Jaranilla J, Petri M. Predictors of self-reported health-related quality of life in systemic lupus erythematosus. Rheumatol Oxf Engl. 2013 Sep;52(9):1651–7.
38. Caramaschi P, Biasi D, Dal Forno I, Adami S. Osteonecrosis in systemic lupus erythematosus: an early, frequent, and not always symptomatic complication. Autoimmune Dis. 2012;2012:725249.
39. Mourão AF, Amaral M, Caetano-Lopes J, Isenberg D. An analysis of joint replacement in patients with systemic lupus erythematosus. Lupus. 2009 Dec;18(14):1298–302.
40. Ehmke TA, Cherian JJ, Wu ES, Jauregui JJ, Banerjee S, Mont MA. Treatment of osteonecrosis in systemic lupus erythematosus: a review. Curr Rheumatol Rep. 2014;16(9):441.
41. Zizic TM, Marcoux C, Hungerford DS, Stevens MB. The early diagnosis of ischemic necrosis of bone. Arthritis Rheum. 1986 Oct;29(10):1177–86.
42. Oh SN, Jee WH, Cho SM, Kim SH, Kang HS, Ryu KN, et al. Osteonecrosis in patients with systemic lupus erythematosus: MR imaging and scintigraphic evaluation. Clin Imaging. 2004 Aug;28(4):305–9.
43. Shigemura T, Nakamura J, Kishida S, Harada Y, Ohtori S, Kamikawa K, et al. Incidence of osteonecrosis associated with corticosteroid therapy among different underlying diseases: Prospective MRI study. Rheumatol Oxf Engl. 2011 Nov;50(11):2023–8.

Skin as a Window to SLE

Avinash Jain

INTRODUCTION

Systemic lupus erythematosus (SLE) is a systemic autoimmune disease affecting multiple organs. Systemic refers to involvement of one to multiple organs as a part of disease process, whereas term *lupus* is a Latin term meaning 'wolf' signifying appearance of rash similar to appearance of a wolf bite. Erythematosus refers to the classical reddening of skin, most commonly face or sun-exposed skin. Skin is an organ where internal disorders are manifested. Impact of any disease on skin, be it localized or generalised, often brings the patient to a health care professional. Cutaneous involvement thus impacts quality of life. Cutaneous involvement can occur in 50–70% of lupus patients. These rashes may precede SLE or may exist independently of lupus or can occur later in the disease course.

Skin involvement in SLE can occur due to multiple reasons and has been classified as lupus specific and lupus non-specific rash[1] (Table 5.1). They are called as lupus specific in view of similar histopathology findings in the form of interface dermatitis except in lupus tumidus and panniculitis. Site, morphology, associated localized and systemic features aid in narrowing down the different subtypes as well as differentials. Annual incidence rate of cutaneous lupus erythematosus (CLE), available from western literature, stands at 2–4.3/100,000 and affects female to male in a ratio of 3:1 to 4:1.[2–5] Higher incidence in males has been reported in the white US population.[6]

Case 1: A 22-year-old young lady comes with the history of erythematous photosensitive rash over cheeks from 6 weeks associated with arthralgia affecting her fingers, wrist and knee. She has been otherwise doing well with no other significant past history. Examination helped in defining the morphology and extent of rash and revealed an erythematous macular rash over face sparing nasolabial folds and upper trunk (Fig. 5.1). There were five tender joints, pallor with no nail/knuckle or mucosal changes to depict nutrient deficiency. Rest of the examination was unremarkable.

TYPES OF RASH

This is a classical rash of lupus called acute cutaneous erythematous (ACLE) which is classified as lupus specific rash (Table 5.1). ACLE rash can be localised or generalized or

Table 5.1: Modified Gilliam classification of SLE rash

SLE specific rash

I. Acute cutaneous lupus erythematosus (ACLE)
   A. Localized ACLE (malar rash)
   B. Generalized ACLE (morbilliform)
   C. Toxic epidermal necrolysis-like ACLE
   D. Bullous LE
II. Subacute cutaneous lupus erythematosus (SCLE)
   A. Annular SCLE
   B. Papulosquamous/psoriasiform
   C. Vesiculobullous annular SCLE
   D. Toxic epidermal necrolysis like SCLE
III. Chronic cutaneous LE (CCLE)
   A. Classic discoid LE (DLE): (a) localized; (b) generalized
   B. Hypertrophic DLE/verrucous DLE
   C. Lupus panniculitis/profundus
   D. Mucosal DLE
   E. LE tumidus
   F. Chilblain LE
   G. Lichenoid DLE (DLE-lichen planus overlap)

SLE non-specific rash

1. Vasculitis
   • Leukocytoclastic vasculitis
   • Polyarteritis nodosa like
   • Vasculopathy
   • Degos disease like
   • Atrophe blanche like
   • Periungal telangiectasia
   • Livedo reticularis
   • Thrombophlebitis
   • Raynaud's phenomenon
   • Erythromelalgia
2. Non-scarring alopecia
   • Lupus hair
   • Telogen effluvium
   • Alopecia areata
3. Sclerodactyly
4. Rheumatoid nodules
5. Calcinosis cutis
6. LE-non-specific bullous lesions
7. Urticaria
8. Papulonodular mucinosis
9. Cutis laxa/anetoderma
10. Acanthosis nigricans (type B insulin resistance)
11. Lichen planus
12. Leg ulcers

may be associated with toxic epidermal necrolysis (TEN) or erythema multiforme major (called Rowell syndrome) in a few cases. This is typically described as erythematous, macular (Table 5.2 for terminology) or maculopapular rash occurring over sun-exposed areas like

Table 5.2: Common terminologies used in description of rash

Type of rash	Morphology	Size	Size more than 10 mm
Macule	A macule is a change in surface color, without elevation or depression	Less 10 mm	Patch
Papule	Circumscribed, solid elevation of skin with no visible fluid	Less than 5–10 mm	Plaque
Vesicle	Circumscribed, fluid-containing, epidermal elevation		Bulla
Nodule	Solid elevated areas of tissue inside or under the skin	0.5–5 cm	Tumor (>5 cm)
Other commonly used terms			
Polycyclic	Two or more connected rings	Polymorphic	Occurring in more than one form
Papulosquamous	Psoriasis like		

malar region, upper torso, forearm and hands. They spare the nasolabial folds and knuckle unlike erythematous rash seen in dermatomyositis which involves nasolabial folds (Figs 5.1–5.2a to c) and knuckles but often spares the phalanges between the inter-phalangeal joints.

They are photosensitive in nature and connote active disease. ACLE rash could be indicative of active internal disease and hence this young lady should also be closely examined for extra-cutaneous signs of disease activity and followed. The rash generally heals without scarring or hyperpigmentation barring in dark skinned individuals where this may leave pigmentation.

Other types of lupus specific rash include subacute cutaneous lupus erythematosus (SCLE) and discoid lupus erythematosus (DLE) or chronic cutaneous lupus erythematosus (CCLE) lesion. Terms acute, subacute or chronic may not necessarily signify duration of disease. These rashes are not mutually exclusive of each other and can occur together. Particularly SCLE rash which can present in two forms that can coexist together or with other types of

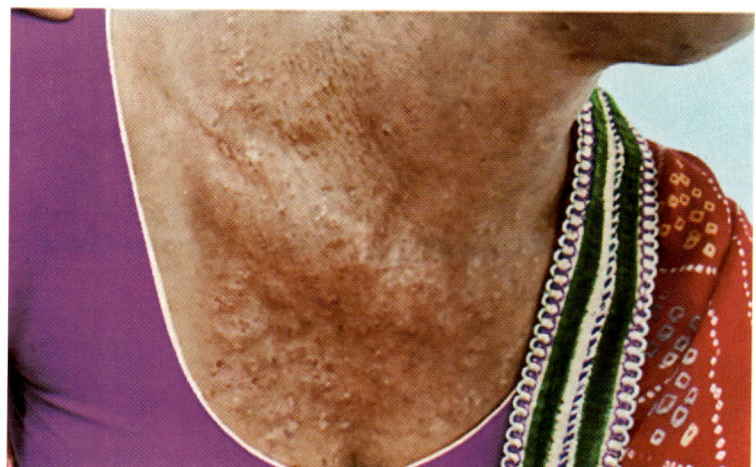

Fig. 5.1: Acute cutaneous lupus erythematosus (ACLE) rash in a patient with lupus. Erythematous maculopapular rash occurring over neck, a sun-exposed area

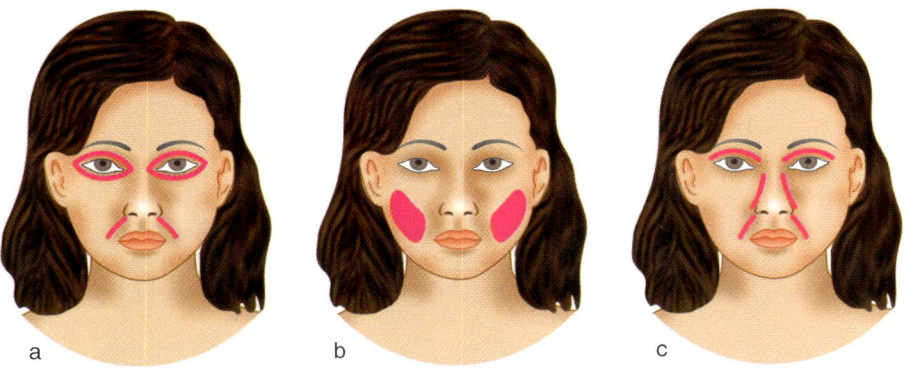

Fig. 5.2a–c: **(a)** Erythematous rash seen in dermatomyositis in a periorbital distribution (heliotrope) and crossing nasolabial folds. **(b)** Hallmark of acute cutaneous erythematous (ACLE) rash is a classical erythematous macular or papular rash occurring over cheeks and bridge of the nose in a symmetric pattern, sparing nasolabial folds, often lasting from weeks to days. **(c)** Erythema with greasy yellow white scale involving nasolabial folds, eyebrows, glabella, and lateral nasal areas in a case of seborrheic dermatitis

lupus rash. Lesions may resemble psoriasis (papulosquamous) or can be annular or polycyclic with peripheral scale and central clearing. Neck, shoulders, extensor surfaces of the arms are archetypally involved. Rarely ACLE or SCLE can have TEN like presentation in the form of an extensive rash affecting the skin and the mucosa.

Table 5.3 highlights the differences amongst the three types of rashes and Table 5.4 compares the prevalence of these rashes in various cohorts across the world.[7–11]

Table 5.3: A comparison of lupus specific rash			
Features	*ACLE*	*SCLE*	*DLE/CCLE*
Description			
Prevalence	60%	10–20%	25%
Erythema	+	+	+
Photosensitivity	+	+	+
Morphology	Macular to papular	Scaly papules Annular Psoriasiform	Erythematous to purplish papule or plaque with induration
Onset and duration	Days to weeks	Weeks to months	Weeks to months
Site	Photo-exposed area	Back, neck, shoulder, extensor surfaces of forearms, spares mid-facial area (under chin)	Both photo-distributed and non-photo-distributed areas Mucosa (mouth, genitalia, conjunctiva, nose)
Types	Localised Generalised	Annular Papulosquamous	Localised Generalised
Sequalae			
Resolution	Complete; temporary hyperpigmentation	May leave hypopigmentation or depigmentation resembling vitiligo	Disfiguring plaque, scar and areas of hypopigmentation with hyperpigmented borders

(Contd...)

Table 5.3: A comparison of lupus specific rash (*Contd...*)

Features	ACLE	SCLE	DLE/CCLE
Scars	Not seen	Generally not seen	Seen
Complication	None	None	Rarely skin malignancy
Autoantibodies		Ro, La (>80%),	U1RNP
Causative drugs	Rare	Hydralazine, ACEi, CCBs, terbinafine	Rare
Differentials	Seborrheic dermatitis Peri-oral dermatitis Acne rosacea Dermatomyositis Acne vulgaris PMLE	Psoriasis *Tinea* Actinic lichen Dermatomyositis Cutaneous T cell lymphoma PMLE	Actinic keratoses Psoriasis vitiligo Basal cell carcinoma

ACLE—acute cutaneous lupus erythematosus; ACE—angiotensin converting enzyme inhibitors; CCB—calcium channel blockers; CCLE—chronic cutaneous lupus erythematosus; DLE—discoid LE; PMLE—polymorphous light eruption; SCLE—subacute cutaneous lupus erythematosus

Table 5.4: Lupus specific rash in different cohorts across the world (expressed as percentage)

	Indian unpublished data	Ribi C, et al.	Rúa-Figueroa Í, et al.	Cervera R, et al.	Györi, et al.
N	466	255	3679	1000	574
ACLE	55.1	41	55.2	58	58
SCLE	15	—	—	—	5.5
DLE	22.7	20	21	10	28

ACLE—acute cutaneous lupus erythematosus; SCLE—subacute cutaneous lupus erythematosus; DLE—discoid LE

Case 2: A 26-year-old, married girl presented to you in a clinic with erythematous plaques with adherent scales over scalp, ear from 2 years. She is worried as she is recently married and wants to know the prognosis and disease progression.

PROGRESSION OF CLE TO SLE

This looks like a typical DLE or CCLE rash (Fig. 5.3) and since it is restricted to above the neck is referred to as localized DLE. Extension of lesions below and above the neck is called as generalized DLE. DLE rash can begin as erythematous or purplish macule or papule or as slightly indurated plaque with adherent scales that extent into dilated hair follicles. Involvement of hair follicles is a prominent feature and occasionally DLE can occur as a butterfly rash sparing nasolabial folds. Other sites that can be affected are mucosal surfaces (mucosal DLE) and non-photoexposed areas. Over time lesion can coalesce to form disfiguring plaques and leave behind scar or areas of hypopigmentation with hyperpigmented borders. Some of these lesions resemble vitiligo.

As far as explaining the prognosis and progression to SLE is concerned, different series, mostly retrospective have described 5–20% of DLE[12–14] can progress to SLE. Features such as generalized DLE, associated arthralgia or arthritis or leucopenia or periungual telangiectasias, raised ESR or abnormal nailfold capillaries may be indirect clues.[15–17] But often these patients have mild systemic features and rarely organ threatening disease.[2,18]

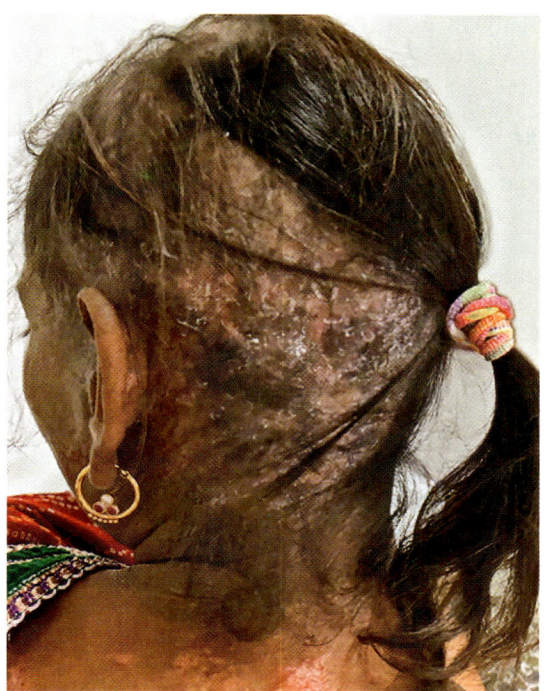

Fig. 5.3: Discoid lupus erythematosus (DLE) rash and associated scarring alopecia seen with DLE

However, up to 25% of SLE patients can have DLE. So, the patient can be reassured, and needs follow-up keeping in mind above systemic features. Serology does not help except patients with high titre ANA may have higher probability of evolving into lupus.[15]

However, ACLE, SCLE rash and non-lupus specific rash are more likely to evolve into lupus. Median time to SLE diagnosis in patients who have cutaneous lupus erythematosus (CLE) is 2.05 years.[5] Probability of diagnosis of SLE after 10 years from CLE is 10–12%[3,5] and 23% after 25 years.[3] Use of hydroxychloroquine has beneficial effect on preventing disease progression as well as major organ involvement.[19]

Amongst the lupus specific rash, lupus tumidus almost never evolves into lupus. Lupus tumidus which lacks immunoglobulin deposition on biopsy, is edematous, indurated and erythematous, seen commonly over cheek (zygomatic arch) and trunk and heals without any sequalae.

Case 3: 50-year-old gentleman was recently diagnosed to have hypertension and has been started on hydrochlorothiazide with good control of blood pressure. He noticed psoriasiform rash over his forearm and upper back with no other systemic findings. What is the probable diagnosis?

DRUG-INDUCED CLE

If you look at the history, one point that is distinctly glaring at you is the onset of rash after starting hydrochlorothiazide. Type of rash and distribution point to the possibility of SCLE type rash. Drug-induced lupus is common in the older age groups beyond 50 years and often presents with fever, rash, arthralgia and serositis with positive anti-histone antibodies and rarely positive anti-dsDNA antibodies. List of drugs definitely implicated include procainamide, hydralazine, minocycline, isoniazid, infliximab, terbinafine, proton pump inhibitors and probable drugs include hydrochlorothiazide, phenytoin, anti-thyroid drugs, sulfasalazine.[20–22] In view of temporal correlation, this gentleman was asked to stop hydrochlorothiazide and switched to amlodipine and tested positive for anti-histone antibodies. Rash disappeared without any need for additional immunosuppression. Median duration from initiation of drug to development of rash is 8 weeks, though the exposure can occur 6 months or longer, prior to diagnosis.[22] Biopsy findings do not differ when compared to SCLE occurring as a part of lupus.[21]

CUTANEOUS DISEASE BEYOND ACLE AND CCLE

Case 4: 22-year-old young lady comes with a history of papules on toes and fingers both in winters and summers. She has no other systemic features but was found to have low leucocyte count. How will you counsel her about diagnosis and probability of having lupus?

The history here is consistent with chilblains, classified as a lupus specific rash (Fig. 5.4). They can occur as papules or plaque or nodule on fingers, toes or even nose and earlobe and may be pruritic to begin with, particularly at onset or in idiopathic type (also referred to as pernio). Chilblain lesions when occurring even in warmer months or associated with Raynaud or DLE or low neutrophil counts and positive autoantibodies are more likely to have lupus. Otherwise, they are commonly seen in winters. This lady needs to be worked up for lupus. Besides a thorough systemic examination, urine routine and ANA by immunofluorescence are advisable.

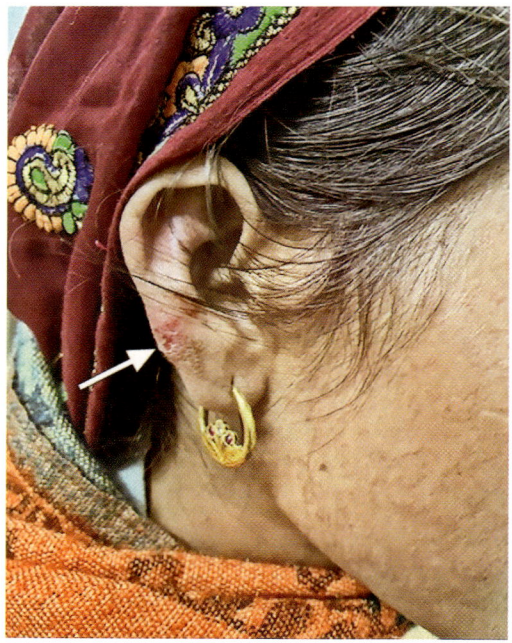

Fig. 5.4: A young lupus patient presented with chilblains (arrow), painful erythematous maculopapular rash over earlobes, which used to get worse in winters

There are various other types of rash described in lupus (Table 5.1). Photosensitivity is defined as abnormal reaction to UV light resulting in cutaneous reaction which persists for hours even after there is no continued exposure to sun.

Lupus panniculitis is inflammation of fat resulting in indurated plaque or depression affecting face, breast, trunk, upper arm, buttock and thigh. If there is an overlying DLE lesion, it is called lupus profundus.

Lichen planus–lupus erythematosus (LP–LE) overlap is characterized by non-photosensitive red–purple colored patch or plaque appearing over extremities. Biopsy and immunofluorescence reveal features of both LP and LE.

SLE patients can also present with palpable purpura or erythematous macular rash over palms and soles which could signify underlying cutaneous vasculitis. It can also present as cutaneous infarcts with areas of ulceration (Fig. 5.5).

Vesiculobullous lesions, urticaria, reticulated palmar erythema and livedo reticularis are some of the other lesions that can be seen in a setting of lupus.

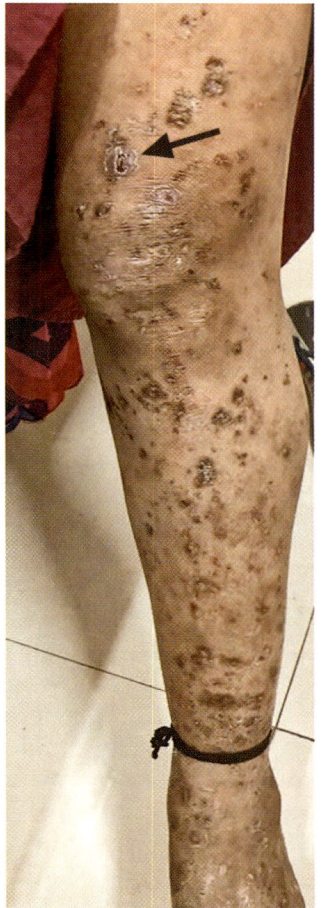

Fig. 5.5: Painful lesions over lower limb in young girl with lupus suggestive of cutaneous vasculitis. There are areas of ulceration and necrosis characterized by blackish discoloration (arrowhead)

Case 5: A 26-year-old lady, known case of lupus from 4 years in view of mucocutaneous (ACLE, oral ulcer), musculoskeletal (polyarthralgia), renal involvement but in remission for 2½ years. She is married and now wishes to conceive and presents to you in OPD with this desire but describes photosensitive malar rash-like she had at onset from last 2 weeks. How will you approach?

SKIN AND DISEASE ACTIVITY

This could be a challenging situation though she only seems to be having a minor flare in form of a cutaneous rash. New onset rash or even a persistent rash in itself means disease activity and is scored as active in disease in activity scores like systemic lupus erythematosus disease activity index (SLEDAI)[23] and British Isles LupusAssessment Group (BILAG).[24] In this situation, it is prudent to assess disease activity in other organs. She was eventually advised to get serology (dsDNA, complements), hemogram, ESR, CRP and urine examination done to assess for disease activity. It is crucial to compare the serology with previous reports as some patients may always have high dsDNA or low complements that may not parallel disease activity. All her reports were normal and she was advised photoprotection using physical barriers like umbrella, clothing particularly use of darker fabrics, UV filters for car, and application of sun protective creams.

For assessing cutaneous disease activity, cutaneous lupus erythematosus disease area and severity index (CLASI) is a good instrument to assess activity (CLASI-A) as well as damage (CLASI-D).[25]

Case 6: A female in her 40s comes with 3 months history of arthralgia and erythematous rash with few papules and telangiectasia over face which gets worse when she is exposed to heat or stressed. There are no other systemic complaints and she has presented to you with ANA 1+ speckled and looks worried.

ALL THAT IS RED IS NOT ACLE: DIFFERENTIAL DIAGNOSIS

Distribution and morphology the rash over the face, including associated arthralgia makes you think immediately about lupus. ANA 1+ could be a red herring here. Her rash gets worsened on exposure to heat or stress, a finding more classical of rosacea. Patients may have burning or stinging sensation that worsened on exposure to heat, stress or extreme temperature, emotional stimuli, hot beverages, spicy food and sun. Typically, central area of the face and nose are affected and can have associated ocular manifestations.

Other differentials that need to be borne in mind in a case of lupus include seborrheic dermatitis; erythematous plaques with greasy yellow white scale over nasolabial folds, eyebrows, glabella, and lateral nasal areas (Fig. 5.2c), perioral dermatitis (steroid rosacea), atopic dermatitis, allergic contact dermatitis and , and erysipelas. All these can mimic ACLE rash. SCLE rash can be confused with Tinea (can be unilateral, sharply demarcated scaling papules), psoriasis or can occur in a setting of paraneoplastic syndrome. Other common mimics include photodermatitis/polymorphous light eruption (pruritic, erythematous, or skin-coloured papules or plaques in a symmetric distribution on sun-exposed skin and may have positive family history), viral exanthem, drug rash, sarcoidosis (lupus pernio, maculopapular rash) or pemphigus or pemphigoid (bullous SLE) or cutaneous malignancy.

Case 7: A 27-year-old female comes with history of erythematous maculopapular eruption over dorsal aspect of forearm, oral ulcer, raised dsDNA, normal C3 and C4 levels and positive ANA on immunofluorescence. She was labelled as lupus, but patient wants to confirm the same by doing a skin biopsy. How relevant is a biopsy in such a case and what will you find?

PATHOLOGY

Biopsy is generally reserved for atypical rash and not required for a typical rash like in this case. Availability of various autoantibodies including lupus specific ones like anti-Smith, anti-ribosomal P have supplanted biopsy. Biopsy reveals interface dermatitis characterised by mononuclear cell infiltrate at the dermal-epidermal junction with basal layer vasculopathic degeneration of keratinocytes, and periadnexal inflammation with varying degrees of follicular plugging and mucin deposition.[26,27] Biopsy may help to differentiate SCLE from DLE as latter has more hyperkeratosis, basement membrane thickening, follicular plugging, inflammatory cells, pilosebaceous atrophy and subepidermal edema.[28,29] Direct immunofluorescence (DIF) reveals immunoglobulin and complement deposition. DIF of non-lesional sun-protected skin is more specific (lupus band test).[30] Bullous lesions too reveal positive DIF but at basement membrane zone.

SKIN AS A WINDOW TO SIDE EFFECTS

Case 8: A 31-year-old lady diagnosed to have lupus in view of ACLE rash, alopecia, and positive ANA and anti-Ro, anti-Sm on immunoblot and was started on hydroxychloroquine, prednisolone 5 mg daily a month ago. She has noticed improvement in her disease manifestations but has noticed pruritic maculopapular rash over chest anteriorly as well as the non-sunexposed areas over forearm and lower back. She denies any non-compliance.

Drug rash can mimic a lupus rash and may add to diagnostic dilemma and increased dose of offending medication(s) mistaking it to be disease activity. Temporal correlation and lack of disease activity elsewhere with normal blood parameters including serology may help. If in doubt, a biopsy may help. This lady was asked to stop hydroxychloroquine and steroid dose was adjusted to 10 mg with addition of anti-histamines. She showed good response with disappearance of this new rash. A number of other cutaneous side effects have been reported with the use of immunosuppressive agents and need to be borne in mind including development of infectious complications like herpes zoster, Tinea, etc. Table 5.5 lists some of the drug-related side effects seen with commonly used medications in lupus.

MANAGEMENT

Management largely depends on the presence or absence of active extra-cutaneous disease activity. For cutaneous lesions, protection from sunlight is a must, which can be achieved using physical barriers as highlighted previously or using sun protection creams. Creams with a higher sun protection factor (SPF) above 50 and preferably above 85 should be used 30 minutes before going out in sun and repeated every 3–4 hours.

Topical therapy in the form of higher potency steroids to begin with, followed by switching over to lesser potent steroids can be effective. Other topical agents available include 0.1% tacrolimus and 0.1% pimecrolimus.[31]

Table 5.5: Drug-related cutaneous side effects	
Drug	*Cutaneous side effects*
Topical steroids	Burning, itching, skin atrophy, steroid rosacea
Hydroxychloroquine	Bleaching of hair, skin and mucosal blue–black pigmentation, acute generalized exanthematous pustulosis, skin erythema, maculopapular rash, urticaria, skin photosensitivity, Steven-Johnson syndrome–toxic epidermal necrolysis (SJS–TEN)
Oral steroids	Thinning of skin, facial erythema, urticaria
Methotrexate	Alopecia, photosensitivity, acne vulgaris, SJS–TEN, urticaria, dyspigmentation, erythema multiforme, furunculosis
Azathioprine	Hypersensitivity, maculopapular rash
Dapsone	Exfoliative dermatitis, morbilliform rash, SJS–TEN, urticaria
Mycopherolate mofetil	Maculopapular rash, ecchymoses, cellulitis
Acitretin	Skin exfoliation, pruritus, skin atrophy

Hydroxychloroquine in a dose of 5 mg/kg is the mainstay of therapy (preferably given as a single dose at night). Yearly ophthalmology screening is recommended after 5 years of therapy unless there are any other risk factors for toxicity like use of tamoxifen or renal failure or prior macular disease.[32] Screening should include fundus examination, automated visual fields plus spectral-domain optical coherence tomography.[32] Baseline fundus examination is also recommended within the first year of starting HCQ.

Other immunosuppressive agents which can be used include chloroquine, quinacrine, prednisolone, methotrexate, mycophenolate, azathioprine, thalidomide, acitretin and for more refractory cases cyclophosphamide, rituximab. Dapsone is effective for bullous LE.

CONCLUSION

Skin involvement is common in lupus and can be the initial presentation. It often reflects active disease and affects quality of life. It is equally essential to keep in mind other mimics and drug-related side effects. Availability of a number of topical and oral medications has improved the outcome.

REFERENCES

1. Gilliam JN, Sontheimer RD. Distinctive cutaneous subsets in the spectrum of lupus erythematosus. J Am Acad Dermatol. 1981 Apr;4(4):471–5.
2. Wallace DJ, Pistiner M, Nessim S, Metzger AL, Klinenberg JR. Cutaneous lupus erythematosus without systemic lupus erythematosus: Clinical and laboratory features. Semin Arthritis Rheum. 1992 Feb;21(4):221–6.
3. Durosaro O, Davis MDP, Reed KB, Rohlinger AL. Incidence of cutaneous lupus erythematosus, 1965-2005: A population-based study. Arch Dermatol. 2009 Mar;145(3):249–53.
4. Grönhagen CM, Fored CM, Granath F, Nyberg F. Cutaneous lupus erythematosus and the association with systemic lupus erythematosus: A population-based cohort of 1088 patients in Sweden. Br J Dermatol. 2011 Jun;164(6):1335–41.
5. Petersen MP, Möller S, Bygum A, Voss A, Bliddal M. Epidemiology of cutaneous lupus erythematosus and the associated risk of systemic lupus erythematosus: A nationwide cohort study in Denmark. Lupus. 2018 Aug;27(9):1424–30.

6. Jarukitsopa S, Hoganson DD, Crowson CS, Sokumbi O, Davis MD, Michet CJ, et al. Epidemiology of systemic lupus erythematosus and cutaneous lupus erythematosus in a predominantly white population in the United States. Arthritis Care Res. 2015 May;67(6):817–28.

7. Jain A, Egambaram M, Chougule A, Parathasarthy J, Sindhu P, Gajula S, et al. Clinical and laboratory features in the first inception cohort of SLE in India: The data of first 466 patients[Abstract]. Indian J Rheumatol. 2019;14(S2):99–249.

8. Györi N, Giannakou I, Chatzidionysiou K, Magder L, van Vollenhoven RF, Petri M. Disease activity patterns over time in patients with SLE: Analysis of the Hopkins Lupus Cohort. Lupus Sci Med. 2017 Feb;4(1):e000192.

9. Cervera R, Khamashta MA, Font J, Sebastiani GD, Gil A, Lavilla P, et al. Systemic lupus erythematosus: Clinical and immunologic patterns of disease expression in a cohort of 1,000 patients. The European Working Party on Systemic Lupus Erythematosus. Medicine (Baltimore). 1993 Mar;72(2):113–24.

10. Ribi C, Trendelenburg M, Gayet-Ageron A, Cohen C, Dayer E, Eisenberger U, et al. The Swiss Systemic lupus erythematosus Cohort Study (SSCS) - cross-sectional analysis of clinical characteristics and treatments across different medical disciplines in Switzerland. Swiss Med Wkly. 2014;144:w13990.

11. Rúa-Figueroa Í, Richi P, López-Longo FJ, Galindo M, Calvo-Alén J, Olivé-Marqués A, et al. Comprehensive description of clinical characteristics of a large systemic lupus erythematosus cohort from the Spanish Rheumatology Society Lupus Registry (RELESSER) with emphasis on complete versus incomplete lupus differences. Medicine (Baltimore). 2015 Jan;94(1):e267.

12. Okon LG, Werth VP. Cutaneous lupus erythematosus: Diagnosis and treatment. Best Pract Res Clin Rheumatol. 2013 Jun;27(3):391–404.

13. Yavuz G, Yavuz I, Bayram I, Aktar R, Bilgili S. Clinic experience in discoid lupus erythematosus: A retrospective study of 132 cases. Adv Dermatol Allergol. 2019;36(6):739–43.

14. Grönhagen CM, Nyberg F. Cutaneous lupus erythematosus?: An update. 2014;5(1).

15. Chong BF, Song J, Olsen NJ. Determining risk factors for developing systemic lupus erythematosus in patients with discoid lupus erythematosus. Br J Dermatol. 2012 Jan;166(1):29–35.

16. Cardinali C, Caproni M, Bernacchi E, Amato L, Fabbri P. The spectrum of cutaneous manifestations in lupus erythematosus—the Italian experience. Lupus. 2000;9(6):417–23.

17. Callen JP. Chronic cutaneous lupus erythematosus. Clinical, laboratory, therapeutic, and prognostic examination of 62 patients. Arch Dermatol. 1982 Jun;118(6):412–6.

18. Wieczorek IT, Propert KJ, Okawa J, Werth VP. Systemic symptoms in the progression of cutaneous to systemic lupus erythematosus. JAMA Dermatol. 2014 Mar;150(3):291–6.

19. James JA, Kim-Howard XR, Bruner BF, Jonsson MK, McClain MT, Arbuckle MR, et al. Hydroxychloroquine sulfate treatment is associated with later onset of systemic lupus erythematosus. Lupus. 2007;16(6):401–9.

20. Chengappa KG. Drug induded lupus. Indian J Rheumatol. 2019;14(5):10–8.

21. Laurinaviciene R, Sandholdt LH, Bygum A. Drug-induced cutaneous lupus erythematosus: 88 new cases. Eur J Dermatol. 2017;27(1):28–33.

22. Grönhagen CM, Fored CM, Linder M, Granath F, Nyberg F. Subacute cutaneous lupus erythematosus and its association with drugs: A population-based matched case-control study of 234 patients in Sweden. Br J Dermatol. 2012 Aug;167(2):296–305.

23. Bombardier C, Gladman DD, Urowitz MB, Caron D, Chang CH, Austin A, et al. Derivation of the sledai. A disease activity index for lupus patients. Arthritis Rheum. 1992;35(6):630–40.

24. Isenberg DA, Rahman A, Allen E, Farewell V, Akil M, Bruce IN, et al. BILAG 2004. Development and initial validation of an updated version of the British Isles Lupus Assessment Group's disease activity index for patients with systemic lupus erythematosus. RheumatolOxf Engl. 2005 Jul;44(7):902–6.

25. Albrecht J, Taylor L, Berlin JA, Dulay S, Ang G, Fakharzadeh S, et al. The CLASI (cutaneous lupus erythematosus disease area and severity index): An outcome instrument for cutaneous lupus erythematosus. J Invest Dermatol. 2005 Nov;125(5):889–94.

26. Provost TT, Reichlin M. Immunopathologic studies of cutaneous lupus erythematosus. J Clin Immunol. 1988 Jul 1;8(4):223–33.

27. Tsokos GC, Lo MS, Reis PC, Sullivan KE. New insights into the immunopathogenesis of systemic lupus erythematosus. Nat Rev Rheumatol. 2016;12(12):716–30.

28. Bangert JL, Freeman RG, Sontheimer RD, Gilliam JN. Subacute cutaneous lupus erythematosus and discoid lupus erythematosus. Comparative histopathologic findings. Arch Dermatol. 1984 Mar;120(3):332–7.
29. Jerdan MS, Hood AF, Moore GW, Callen JP. Histopathologic comparison of the subsets of lupus erythematosus. Arch Dermatol. 1990 Jan;126(1):52–5.
30. Reich A, Marcinow K, Bialynicki-Birula R. The lupus band test in systemic lupus erythematosus patients. Ther Clin Risk Manag. 2011;7:27–32.
31. Jessop S, Whitelaw DA, Grainge MJ, Jayasekera P. Drugs for discoid lupus erythematosus. Cochrane Database Syst Rev. 2017 05;5:CD002954.
32. Marmor MF, Kellner U, Lai TY, Melles RB, Mieler WF; American Academy of Ophthalmology. Recommendations on screening for chloroquine and hydroxychloroquine retinopathy (2016 Revision). Ophthalmology. 2016 Jun;123(6):1386–94.

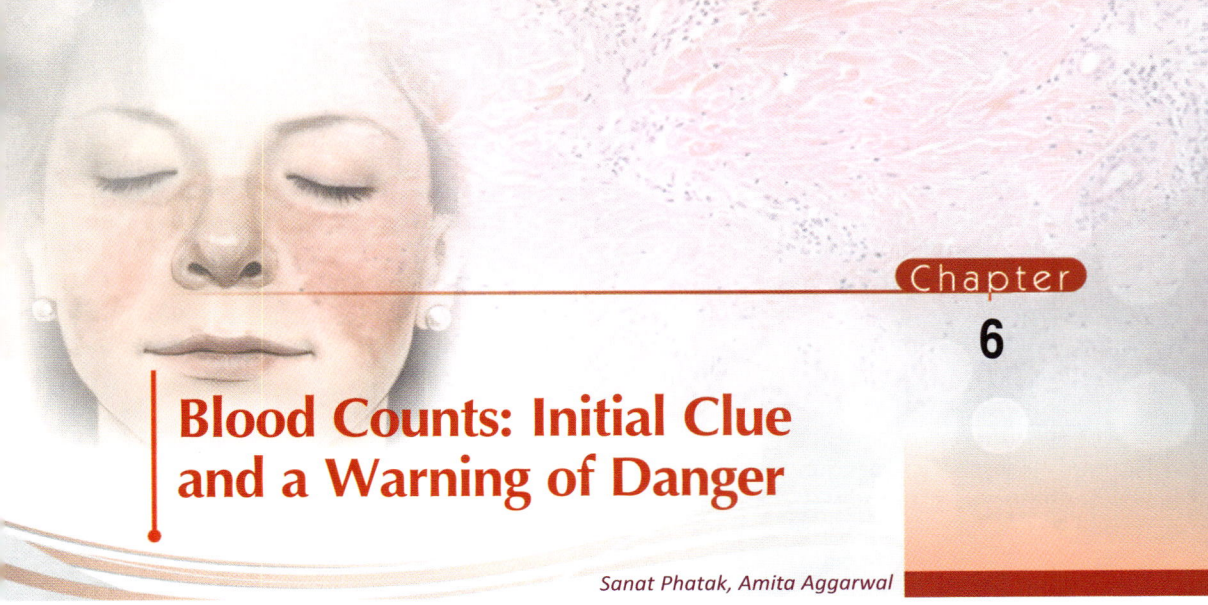

Blood Counts: Initial Clue and a Warning of Danger

Sanat Phatak, Amita Aggarwal

INTRODUCTION

Hematological abnormalities are common in SLE and each type of blood cell can be involved. The spectrum of manifestations ranges from life-threatening hemolysis to incidental laboratory abnormalities. Consequently, they figure prominently in classification criteria, with the recent SLICC criteria allotting 3 of 11 clinical criteria to them.[1] While a large percentage of patients with SLE show hematological abnormalities, they need not necessarily signify disease activity—drug-related marrow suppression, infection and sepsis, complications, comorbidities, secondary malignancy and co-existent nutrient deficiencies are all important considerations. Looking closely at the blood cell counts—namely leucocyte and platelet—can provide valuable information about the disease status. In some scenarios, changes in blood counts may herald the onset of life-threatening manifestations in lupus and offer an opportunity to intervene early. The hemogram is a simple and widely available test and does not need specialized equipment. We discuss cytopenias in lupus considering a few commonly encountered clinical scenarios.

Case 1: A 37-year-old lady had fatigue and diffuse muscle ache for 2 years. On inquiring, she also had Raynaud's phenomenon in winters. All her lab investigations done were reported to be normal. She received vitamin B_{12}, iron and vitamin D. Later a diagnosis of fibromyalgia was made, but she did not have benefit from pregabalin or duloxetine. Now she presented with pedal edema and new onset hypertension for the past 1 month. Labs showed a positive ANA and active urinary sediment with RBCs, WBCs and casts. Anti dsDNA antibodies were positive. Kidney biopsy demonstrated class III lupus nephritis; oral steroids and mycophenolate mofetil were initiated. A review of multiple previous investigations demonstrated a low normal leucocyte count (in the range of 3900 and 4500/mm³) with low absolute lymphocyte count (390–700).

LYMPHOPENIA

This patient presented with Frank lupus nephritis, but had non-specific symptoms for 2 years prior to the major organ involvement. In retrospect, all her reports show lymphopenia, which was attributed to other causes. Lymphopenia is a hallmark of the blood picture of SLE and may be the first clue to the diagnosis of the disease. Most classification criteria of

SLE define lymphopenia as an absolute lymphocyte count of less than 1500/mm³.[1] The clinical relevance of lymphopenia is indeterminate. Studies, including one from India, demonstrated an increased infection risk in patients with lymphopenia.[2] In contrast, studies from the west have not found an effect on infection rate or on patient survival.[3] Lymphopenia does associate with lupus disease activity in general, and musculoskeletal, systemic and nervous manifestations in particular.[4] Therefore, it is difficult to ascertain whether the increased infection risk found in the patients can be attributed to depressed protective immunity by bloodstream lymphocytes, or to the higher doses of immunosuppressive (IS) drugs that this group of patients receives.

The presence of lymphopenia alone does not need specific treatment, and is likely to resolve with IS treatment given for other indications. Some authors recommend Pneumocystis prophylaxis in patients with very low lymphocyte counts—with the caveat that TMP–SMX may suppress blood counts further.[5] Lymphocyte numbers are a useful tool as a biomarker of lupus disease activity and dropping counts herald disease relapse. A patient with new onset lymphopenia found routinely on follow up justifies closer follow up for subsequent flare.[6]

Case 2: A 14-year-old girl has seizures, malar rash and class III lupus nephritis and was started on monthly IV pulse cyclophosphamide (CYC) pulses along with prednisolone. She returned 12 days after her second pulse with fever, productive cough and breathlessness; a chest X-ray revealed a patch in right lower zone. Due to hypoxemia she was admitted to the hospital for IV antibiotics. Blood reports showed a leucocyte count of 1800 (30% neutrophils and 70% lymphocytes). Platelet count, liver functions and creatinine were normal. Infection resolved with 7 days of hospital stay and neutrophil counts at discharge were 3000/mm³.

NEUTROPENIA

This girl presented with a severe chest infection in the setting of neutropenia. The definition of neutropenia is generally considered to be a neutrophil count of <1500 cells/cu mm, although definitions vary; the WHO defines neutropenia when TLC is <1800 m³.[7] Considering the temporal relationship with the IV cyclophosphamide, the leucopenia in this case is most likely attributable to the drug. Cyclophosphamide is an alkylating agent and is associated with dose dependent neutropenia and leucopenia. The nadir WBC count is expected at an interval of 8–14 days following the CYC pulse.[8] A WBC nadir of less than 3000/mm³ is associated with a higher infection rate and mandates dose reduction in subsequent pulses.[9] Oral CYC is associated with a higher degree of both cytopenia as well as infection risk, possibly owing to higher cumulative dosages. Apart from CYC, up to one-fourth of patients receiving azathioprine (AZA) get dose dependent leucopenia. Nearly 10% of patients have reduced activity of the enzyme thiopurine methyltransferase (TPMT), but only 0.3% have very low activity which results in an accumulation of thioguanine metabolites, cytotoxic to hematologic cells.[10] Azathioprine-induced leucopenia most commonly occurs between 4 to 10 weeks of starting the drug, and in the absence of the availability of TPMT testing it is advisable to start at a lower dose.[11]

Neutropenia can be associated with SLE itself; a case series found that 5% SLE patients had moderate to severe neutropenia; all of which could not be explained by drug-related myelosuppression.[12] The pathogenesis of neutropenia in SLE is most commonly reduced survival of neutrophils; circulating complement-activating anti-neutrophil antibodies have been demonstrated.[13] However, granulocytemonocyte colony formation was also deficient in SLE, which probably adds to the problem.[14,15] Patients with anti-Ro antibodies are more likely to get neutropenia, due to cross-reactivity of Ro antigen with a neutrophil surface antigen.[15] Glucocorticoids increase neutrophil counts due to increased margination and may mask an underlying neutropenia.[16]

Case 3: A 10-year-old boy diagnosed with SLE was doing well on low dose steroid and hydroxychloroquine. He presented with new onset high grade fever without any obvious respiratory, urinary or abdominal focus. There had only been a history of upper respiratory tract infection a week prior to this fever. After 2 days of his fever his mother noticed a yellowish tinge to his eyes. He also developed purpuric region on his trunk and wrist. His friends thought his concentration is lower than usual; he also complained of headache. Empirical oral antibiotics do not help. Investigations demonstrated Hb 7.8, leucopenia (TLC 3300, ANC 1000/mm³), platelets 40000/mm³. Liver enzymes were raised (AST 440 IU, ALT 520 IU/L) and prothrombin time was deranged (INR 3.0). Further investigations revealed a serum ferritin of 1600 ug/dL and bone marrow aspirate showed hemophagocytosis. IV methylprednisolone was initiated, and cytopenias started improving on day 2. Fever settled with the treatment, and cyclophosphamide was commenced.

MACROPHAGE ACTIVATION SYNDROME

This boy with SLE came with a severe, multisystem complication—with cytopenia, coagulopathy and liver involvement, temporally connected to an episode of preceding infection. Macrophage activation syndrome (MAS) is caused by an abnormal hyper-activation of macrophages and T lymphocytes.[17] Macrophages demonstrate hemophagocytic activity, as was seen in the bone marrow in this patient. The major manifestations of this syndrome are believed to occur as a result of overproduction of cytokines and a resultant hyperinflammatory state.[18] Coagulopathy and extremely high levels of ferritin are characteristics of MAS. MAS occurring in autoimmune diseases such as SLE, Kawasaki disease and systemic onset juvenile idiopathic arthritis (SJIA) is considered 'secondary' hemophagocytic lymphohistiocytosis (HLH), where the abnormalities in the cytolytic pathways are acquired, in contrast to being genetically inherited in 'primary' HLH.[19] A preceding infection (especially viral, such as CMV) is commonly present. Prolonged high-grade fever, worsening cytopenia in a sick patient should prompt consideration of the diagnosis. Detection in the setting of SLE is more challenging than in SJIA as cytopenia, fever, lymphadenopathy, CNS involvement and liver dysfunction can be a manifestation of disease activity itself. In a case series of MAS in juvenile SLE, one-third patients did not fulfill the 2004 HLH criteria—compelling the authors to describe SLE specific diagnostic guidelines for MAS.[20] MAS in SLE has a higher frequency of cardiac involvement and lower frequency of hepatosplenomegaly[21] Patients with MAS generally have more active disease with a higher SLEDAI and higher CRP values.[22] MAS in the context of SLE rarely warrants therapy with etoposide containing regimens used in primary HLH as most patients do well with intensification of immunosuppressive therapy including IV pulses with steroid, cyclophosphamide and other drugs.[20]

Case 4: A 50-year-old asymptomatic woman was found to have a platelet count of 80,000/mm³ on routine evaluation. She had no history of any bleeding. Over the subsequent 6 months, she received therapy with vitamin B$_{12}$, however, her platelet counts dropped to 50,000/mm³. Hemoglobin and leucocyte counts were normal. A bone marrow aspiration demonstrated increased megakaryopoiesis. Serology for chronic viral infections (HIV, HCV) were negative. ANA was positive with a speckled pattern on immunofluorescence. The platelet counts improved with steroids, and were tapered off over 4 months. 1 year after this presentation, she developed a malar rash and pedal edema; urine routine showed nephritic sediment.

THROMBOCYTOPENIA

This case highlights that isolated thrombocytopenia (TCP) due to peripheral destruction being diagnosed as ITP may be the initial symptom of SLE. More than one-tenth of patients with isolated ITP evolved into SLE in a case series, and thus follow-up is important.[23] The megakaryocyte destruction is believed to be autoantibody mediated: Antiplatelet antibodies are found in most patients.[24] Though these are not routinely tested. The antibody specificity differs from 'native' ITP: Platelet glycoproteins (Gp IIb/IIIa, Ib/IX) are rarely targeted in SLE associated TCP[25] Antiphospholipid antibodies are also associated with TCP in SLE, conferring a risk ratio of 4. Chronic TCP in SLE is rarely severe enough to cause life-threatening bleeding manifestations. However, TCP is associated with disease activity in other organs, viz. renal, neurological and autoimmune hemolytic anemia.[26] Unlike lymphopenia, thrombocytopenia is independently associated with a worse prognosis and a higher likelihood of death. Treatment modalities are dictated by severity of TCP. Mild to moderate TCP does not warrant any specific treatment and can be observed. Physicians treat TCP if counts are less than 50000/mm^3 or associated with clinical bleeding. SLE-related TCP responds well to glucocorticoids with nearly 80% achieving remission with oral prednisolone alone. However, relapses are common and sustained remission is seen only in 20% in the years following GC withdrawal, making the case for a steroid sparing agent.[27] Various agents, including AZA, mycophenolate, danazol and cyclosporine have been used. Recent observational studies demonstrate efficacy of B cell depletion therapy with rituximab in resistant thrombocytopenia.[28] In acute life-threatening cases, intravenous immunoglobulin (IVIg) infusion has been useful. Unlike ITP, splenectomy is generally avoided in SLE, owing to the increased risk of life-threatening infections including staphylococcal and pneumococcal sepsis and death in these immunosuppressed patients.[29]

Case 5: A 25-year-old lady with known SLE for 3 years, hitherto involving only joints and skin, presented in her post-partum period after having delivered a small for age infant 3 months ago. She had fever for 5 days which did not respond to paracetamol and became drowsy for 48 hours prior to admission. She also developed new onset pedal edema. Blood pressure was 180/110 mm Hg. She was drowsy but had no focal neurological deficits. Hemogram showed anemia, leukocytosis and platelet counts of 15000/mm^3. Reticulocyte count was high. Biochemical tests showed creatinine 3.2 mg/dl, total bilirubin of 3 mg/dl with 60% indirect bilirubin. Urine examination showed no active sediment. A careful examination of the peripheral smear showed 6% schistocytes. Lactate dehydrogenase (LDH) levels were 7 times upper limit normal. She was initiated on plasma exchange (PLEX), and sensorium improved over 2 days, platelet counts normalized after 16 days of daily PLEX.

MICROANGIOPATHIC HEMOLYTIC ANEMIA

This patient presented with neurological symptoms along with laboratory evidence of TCP and intravascular microangiopathic hemolysis (MAHA). Fulfillment of the 'pentad' of manifestations including renal injury and neurological symptoms indicate thrombotic thrombocytopenic purpura (TTP).[30] Unexplained MAHA in a patient fulfilling ACR criteria of SLE is termed SLE–TTP.[31] Descriptions of this rare but life-threatening manifestation remain limited to case series and case reports. Owing to high rate of mortality in patients who do not receive timely treatment, recognizing this entity is important in clinical practice. TTP is characterized by the deficiency of the metalloproteinase ADAMTS13, which leads to the formation of intravascular nets of vWF multimers and consequent hemolysis. In contrast

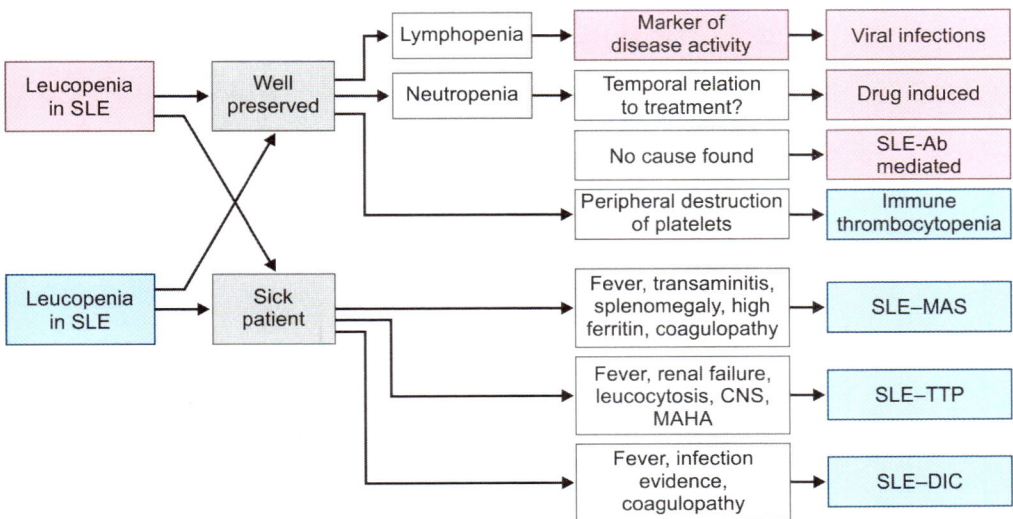

Fig. 6.1: Approach to cytopenia in a patient with systemic lupus erythematosus (SLE). A consideration of the cell type affected and clinical status of the patient helps in informing the differential diagnosis, along with specific investigations

to TTP, nearly three-fourths of patients with SLE–TTP have normal ADAMTS levels, suggesting different pathogenetic mechanisms.[32] Autoantibodies to ADAMTS13 have been demonstrated.[33] Direct endothelial activation and complement mediated endothelial damage have also been hypothesized. Drugs used in SLE such as tacrolimus and cyclosporine may precipitate TTP. Unlike most of the other hematological manifestations, TTP does not necessarily correlate with disease activity. Plasma exchange is successful and has revolutionized outcomes in SLE–TTP just as in TTP.[32] In a case series, plasma exchange was found to be better than plasmapheresis alone, suggesting that plasma infusion may have an additional benefit by overwhelming antibodies to ADAMTS13. Studies have demonstrated a higher mortality in SLE–TTP than TTP, however most of these come from a pre-plasmapheresis era—and probably owe to the added morbidity of the underlying disease. A more recent case series from Singapore also showed that SLE–TTP tended to be more aggressive as compared to TTP; however the mortality rates were similar.[34] Immuno-suppression, with pulsed IV glucocorticoids, cyclophosphamide and mycophenolate have also been found to be useful, unlike in TTP.[35]

These cases demonstrate the wide variety of hematological entities that can be diagnosed in SLE, just by looking at blood cell counts. It is useful to consider which blood lines are affected, and how sick the patient is. Along with associated clinical features, these help in arriving at a diagnosis (Fig. 6.1). As management of each condition differs, it is important to have a high index of suspicion for each condition, especially those that can progress to life-threatening disease.

REFERENCES

1. Petri M, Orbai AM, Alarcón GS, Gordon C, Merrill JT, Fortin PR, et al. Derivation and validation of the systemic lupus international collaborating clinics classification criteria for systemic lupus erythematosus. Arthritis Rheum. 2012;64:2677–86.

2. Bhuyar U, Malaviya A. Deficiency of T cells in blood and tissues and severity of infections in systemic lupus erythematosus. Ind J Med Res. 1978;67:269–78.
3. Sultan S, Begum S, Isenberg D. Prevalence, patterns of disease and outcome in patients with systemic lupus erythematosus who develop severe haematological problems. Rheumatology. 2003;42:230–4.
4. Isenberg DA, Patterson KG, Todd-Pokropek A, Snaith ML, Goldstone AH. Haematological aspects of systemic lupus erythematosus: A reappraisal using automated methods. Acta haematologica. 1982;67:242–8.
5. Keser G, Sequeira J, Khamashta MA, Hughes GR. Anti-Ro and lymphopenia in SLE. Lupus. 1993;2:63.
6. Rivero SJ, Díaz-Jouanen E, Alarcón? Segovia D. Lymphopenia in systemic lupus erythematosus. Arthritis Rheum. 1978;21:295–305.
7. Valent P. Low blood counts: immune mediated, idiopathic, or myelodysplasia. ASH Education Program Book. 2012;2012:485–91.
8. Fraiser LH, Kanekal S, Kehrer JP. Cyclophosphamide toxicity. Drugs. 1991;42:781–95.
9. Pryor BD, Bologna SG, Kahl LE. Risk factors for serious infection during treatment with cyclophosphamide and high-dose corticosteroids for systemic lupus erythematosus. Arthritis Rheum. 1996;39:1475–82.
10. Woodson L, Dunnette JH, Weinshilboum RM. Pharmacogenetics of human thiopurine methyltransferase: Kidney-erythrocyte correlation and immunotitration studies. J Pharmacol Exp Ther. 1982;222:174–81.
11. Belmont M. Pharmacology and side effects of azathioprine when used in rheumatic diseases. Waltham: UpToDate. 2015.
12. Martinez-Banos D, Crispin J, Lazo-Langner A, Sánchez-Guerrero J. Moderate and severe neutropenia in patients with systemic lupus erythematosus. Rheumatology. 2006;45:994–8.
13. Starkebaum G, Price TH, Lee MY, Arend WP. Autoimmune neutropenia in systemic lupus erythematosus. Arthritis Rheum. 1978;21:504–12.
14. Matsuyama W, Yamamoto M, Higashimoto I, Oonakahara K-i, Watanabe M, Machida K, et al. TNF-related apoptosis-inducing ligand is involved in neutropenia of systemic lupus erythematosus. Blood. 2004;104:184–91.
15. Kurien B, Newland J, Paczkowski C, Moore K, Scofield R. Association of neutropenia in systemic lupus erythematosus (SLE) with anti-Ro and binding of an immunologically cross-reactive neutrophil membrane antigen. Clin Exp Immunol. 2000;120:209–17.
16. Sugimoto T, Soumura M, Tanaka Y, Uzu T, Nishio Y, Kashiwagi A. Early morning neutropenia in a patient with systemic lupus erythematosus. Mod Rheumatol. 2006;16:267–8.
17. Grom AA, Horne A, De Benedetti F. Macrophage activation syndrome in the era of biologic therapy. Nat Rev Rheumatol. 2016;12:259.
18. Sawhney S, Woo P, Murray K. Macrophage activation syndrome: a Potentially fatal complication of rheumatic disorders. Arch Dis Child. 2001;85:421–6.
19. Stephan J, Kone-Paut I, Galambrun C, Mouy R, Bader-Meunier B, Prieur AM. Reactive haemophagocytic syndrome in children with inflammatory disorders. A retrospective study of 24 patients. Rheumatology. 2001;40:1285–92.
20. Parodi A, Daví S, Pringe AB, Pistorio A, Ruperto N, Magni-Manzoni S, et al. Macrophage activation syndrome in juvenile systemic lupus erythematosus: a multinational multicenter study of thirty-eight patients. Arthritis Rheum. 2009;60:3388–99.
21. Lambotte O, Khellaf M, Harmouche H, Bader-Meunier B, Manceron V, Goujard C, et al. Characteristics and long-term outcome of 15 episodes of systemic lupus erythematosus-associated hemophagocytic syndrome. Medicine. 2006;85:169–82.
22. Kim J-M, Kwok S-K, Ju JH, Kim H-Y, Park S-H. Reactive hemophagocytic syndrome in adult Korean patients with systemic lupus erythematosus: a case-control study and literature review. J Rheumatol. 2012;39:86–93.
23. Mestanza-Peralta M, Ariza-Ariza R, Cardiel M, Alcocer-Varela J. Thrombocytopenic purpura as initial manifestation of systemic lupus erythematosus. J Rheumatol. 1997;24:867–70.
24. Howe S, Lynch D. Platelet antibody binding in systemic lupus erythematosus. J Rheumatol. 1987;14:482–6.

25. Fabris F, Casonato A, Randi ML, Luzzatto G, Girolami A. Clinical significance of surface and internal pools of platelet-associated immunoglobulins in immune thrombocytopenia. Scand J Haematol. 1986;37:215–20.
26. Miller MH, Urowitz MB, Gladman DD. The significance of thrombocytopenia in systemic lupus erythematosus. Arthritis Rheum. 1983;26:1181–6.
27. Arnal C, Piette J-C, Léone J, Taillan B, Hachulla E, Roudot-Thoraval F, et al. Treatment of severe immune thrombocytopenia associated with systemic lupus erythematosus: 59 cases. J Rheumatol. 2002;29:75–83.
28. Matsubara K, Takahashi Y, Hayakawa A, Tanaka F, Nakadate H, Sakai M, et al. Long-term follow-up of children with refractory immune thrombocytopenia treated with rituximab. Int J Hematol. 2014;99:429–36.
29. Alarcon-Segovia D. Splenectomy has a limited role in the management of lupus with thrombocytopenia. J Rheumatol. 2002;29:1–2.
30. Zheng XL, Sadler JE. Pathogenesis of thrombotic microangiopathies. Annu Rev path Mech Dis. 2008; 3:249–77.
31. Blum D, Blake G. Lupus-associated thrombotic thrombocytopenic purpura-like microangiopathy. World J Nephrol. 2015;4:528.
32. Matsuyama T, Kuwana M, Matsumoto M, Isonishi A, Inokuma S, Fujimura Y. Heterogeneous pathogenic processes of thrombotic microangiopathies in patients with connective tissue diseases. Thrombosis and haemostasis. 2009;101:371–8.
33. Changcharoen B, Bolger Jr DT. Case Report: Thrombotic thrombocytopenic purpura as an initial presentation of systemic lupus erythematosus with acquired ADAMTS13 antibody. BMJ case reports. 2015;2015.
34. Letchumanan P, Ng H-J, Lee L-H, Thumboo J. A comparison of thrombotic thrombocytopenic purpura in an inception cohort of patients with and without systemic lupus erythematosus. Rheumatology. 2009;48:399–403.
35. Hamasaki K, Mimura T, Kanda H, Kubo K, Setoguchi K, Satoh T, et al. Systemic lupus erythematosus and thrombotic thrombocytopenic purpura: A case report and literature review. Clin Rheumatol. 2003;22(4-5):355–8.

Nephritis: The Major Challenge in Lupus

Rudrarpan Chatterjee, Amita Aggarwal

INTRODUCTION

Systemic lupus erythematosus (SLE) is a multisystem disease and renal involvement is one of the most important determinants of outcome in SLE. Renal involvement can lead to a variety of pathological changes: glomerulonephritis, interstitial nephritis, anti-phospholipid antibody-associated nephropathy or renal vein thrombosis, thrombotic microangiopathy, etc. Similarly, the clinical manifestations can also be varied from asymptomatic disease to acute renal failure.

Case 1: A 25-year-old lady presents with malar rash, polyarthralgia, fever and right sided pleural effusion. Investigations reveal anemia, thrombocytopenia, ANA positivity and low complements. Urine examination shows ++ proteinuria, 7–10 RBCs/high power field and hyaline casts. 24-hour urine protein excretion is 2.1 grams. Serum creatinine is 0.8 mg/dl and anti-dsDNA antibodies are >300 IU. This case illustrates that renal involvement can be totally asymptomatic and every patient with lupus should have a urine examination.

PREVALENCE

The prevalence of lupus nephritis is variable depending on age, ethnicity and use of renal biopsy. A recent systematic review and meta-analysis of 5 studies with 2781 patients found prevalence of biopsy proven LN to vary from 16.9 to 42.8%. The overall prevalence was 29% (95% CI 20–38%).[1] A higher prevalence of 50–60% was found in Asian populations.[2] Lupus nephritis is a known predictor of mortality in the first decade of the disease and is second only to infections in our country. As lupus affects young child bearing population it is a significant contributor to disease adjusted life years lost.

CLINICAL FEATURES

Lupus nephritis may present with only asymptomatic urinary abnormality or can present acutely as rapidly progressive renal failure (Table 7.1).[3] A good urine analysis with special emphasis on cells and cellular casts can help in early diagnosis of LN. All patients of SLE should be screened for nephritis at the initial diagnosis. If urine examination is normal at

Table 7.1: Clinical features of lupus nephritis	
Clinical feature	*Prevalence (%)*
Proteinuria	100
Nephrotic range proteinuria/nephrotic syndrome	50
Microscopic hematuria	80
Macroscopic hematuria	05
Urinary red blood cell casts	30
Other urinary cellular casts	30
Renal insufficiency	60
Rapidly progressive renal failure	15
Hypertension	30
Tubular abnormalities	70

onset, regular follow-up 6–12 monthly is needed for any fresh evidence of LN. In a large (N = 1827) multicentric and multiethnic cohort of patients of SLE, LN was present in 38.1% out of whom 80.9% had LN at diagnosis.[4]

RENAL BIOPSY IN A PATIENT WITH SLE

Though renal biopsy is an invasive process it is an important tool in the management of LN. It provides evidence of severity of active glomerular disease as well as chronic changes which have bearing on long-term outcome of LN. Though there are others, who believe that with the progress in immunosuppressive therapies, a renal biopsy may not be necessary at onset of LN in patients in whom urine analysis reveals active urinary sediments.[5] In addition to providing information about LN, biopsy can also help in diagnosing pathologies other than lupus nephritis. In a study of 200 patients with SLE, 5% of patients had other diagnoses like IgA nephropathy, IgM nephropathy, thin basement membrane disease, minimal change disease and focal segmental glomerulosclerosis etc.[6]

Lupus podocytopathy, characterized by minimal changes on light microscopy and a severe effacement of podocytes on electron microscopy, is an entity that has recently come into common clinical parlance and can only be confirmed on a renal biopsy.[7,8] This has direct implications on management of these patients.

Immunofluorescence microscopy in LN typically shows a full house pattern, that is deposition of IgG, IgM, IgA, C3 and C1q. This is helpful in distinguishing proliferative lupus nephritis from other proliferative glomerulonephritis.

Different society guidelines are available on when to renal biopsy. The two commonly used guidelines are given in Table 7.2.[9,10] While EULAR-ERA-EDTA guidelines recommend biopsy within a month of diagnosis and before start of immunosuppressive therapy, the American College of Rheumatology (ACR) recommend it at any time. Delay in renal biopsy has been linked to poor outcome in some studies.

Case 2: A 28-year-old lady was diagnosed with SLE in 2015 when she had rash, polyarthralgias, serositis and hypertension. Urine analysis showed 1.36 g proteinuria and active urinary sediments. A kidney biopsy revealed Class IV nephritis with activity index of 7/24 and chronicity index of 0/12 (Fig. 7.1), She was treated with MMF and achieved remission. She stopped treatment on her own after 3 years and now presented with pedal edema. Urine examination showed microscopic hematuria with proteinuria of 1.2 g. Repeat kidney biopsy revealed class IV nephritis with cellular crescents in 6/15 glomeruli. Her activity index was 6/24 and chronicity index was 2/12.

Table 7.2: Indications for renal biopsy at onset of lupus nephritis

EULAR-ERA-EDTA guidelines (2012)	ACR guidelines (2012)
≥500 mg/day proteinuria	≥1 g/day proteinuria
Glomerular hematuria/cellular casts	≥500 mg/day proteinuria with hematuria
Deranged renal function	≥5 RBC's/high power field
	≥500 mg/day proteinuria with cellular casts

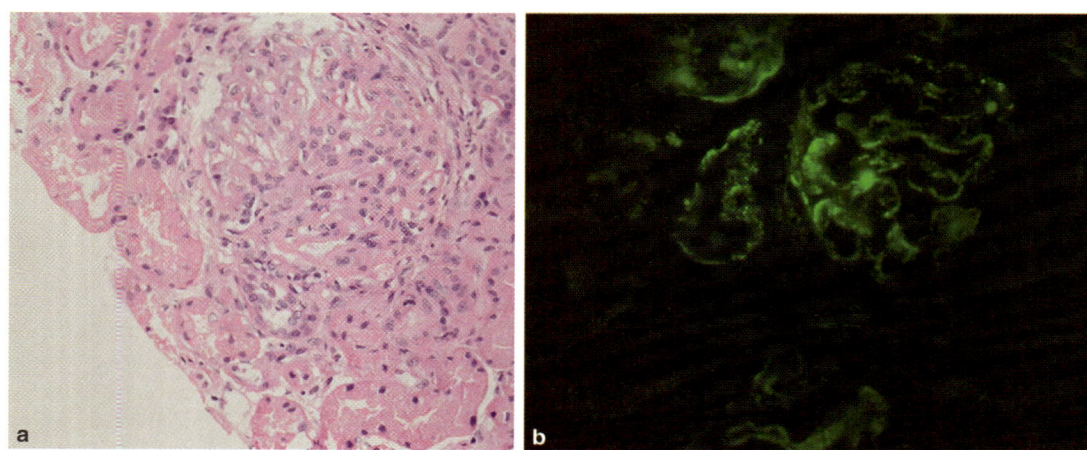

Fig. 7.1a and b: (a) Kidney biopsy showing an enlarged glomerulus with endocapillary proliferation involving the whole glomerulus. **(b)** Immunofluorescence study shows granular deposits of IgG in the glomerulus of a patient with class IV lupus nephritis

The indications for a repeat renal biopsy are equally contentious. Per protocol biopsies at the end of the maintenance phase of therapy to decide regarding discontinuation of treatment can be justified by the fact that lupus nephritis may be active even after years of immune-suppression and may lead to chronic kidney disease if therapy is stopped.[5] An alternate argument is that persistent histological abnormalities may be seen even in those without any ongoing systemic immune injury and immune deposits may persist for several months without disease activity.[11]

The other indication for repeat biopsy is lupus nephritis flare. Nearly two-thirds of patients with class II LN in the first biopsy and 43% with class V may show transition to class III or IV.[12] This requires a switch to more potent immunosuppression. Thus, renal biopsy is indicated in all patients with recent onset LN, nephritic flare or failure to achieve remission during therapy.

Renal Histology

All biopsies should be processed for routine light microscopy and immunofluorescence study. Further, any patient with isolated nephrotic range proteinuria should also have electron microscopy evaluation to rule out lupus podocytopathy.[13]

The ISN/RPS classification of lupus nephritis was initially proposed in 2004 and has recently been modified by a consensus committee.[14] The major changes are summarized here (Table 7.3).

Table 7.3: The modified ISN/RPN classification of lupus nephritis

Class	Characteristic features	Modifications
Class I: Minimal mesangial lupus nephritis	Normal glomeruli by light microscopy, but mesangial immune deposits by immunofluorescence.	
Class II: Mesangial proliferative lupus nephritis	Active or inactive focal, segmental or global endo- or extracapillary glomerulonephritis involving ≤50% of all glomeruli, typically with focal subendothelial immune deposits, with or without mesangial alterations.	Mesangial hypercellularity has been clearly defined as 4 or more nuclei surrounded by matrix in the mesangial region excluding the hilar region.
Class III: Focal proliferative lupus nephritis.	Active or inactive focal, segmental or global endo- or extracapillary glomerulonephritis involving ≤50% of all glomeruli, typically with focal sub-endothelial immune deposits, with or without mesangial alterations.	Endocapillary proliferation has been replaced by the term endocapillary hypercellularity. The A/C/AC designations of class III and IV have been removed and replaced by definition of the NIH activity and chronicity index. Activity is scored on a scale of 0–24 whereas chronicity is scored on a scale of 0–12.
Class IV: Diffuse proliferative lupus nephritis.	Active or inactive diffuse, segmental or global endo- or extracapillary glomerulonephritis involving ≥50% of all glomeruli, typically with diffuse subendothelial immune deposits, with or without mesangial alterations.	The segmental (S) and global (G) designations of class IV lupus nephritis have been removed. Crescents have been defined and classified as celluar, fibrocellular and fibrous. Definitions for adhesions and fibrinoid necrosis have been included. Interstitial inflammation, fibrosis and vascular thrombosis to be reported separately.
Class V: Membranous lupus nephritis	Global or segmental subepithelial immune deposits or their morphologic sequelae by light microscopy and by immunofluorescence or electron microscopy, with or without mesangial alterations.	
Class VI: Advanced sclerotic lupus nephritis	≥90% of glomeruli globally sclerosed without residual activity.	

The inclusion of type of crescent and interstitial fibrosis in the description of biopsies gives a fare idea about the severity and chronicity of the lesions and may help decide the prognosis as well as influence how aggressively we treat our patients. In the clinic the semiquantitative descriptions of activity and chronicity as per the modified NIH activity and chronicity index[15] is highly useful as it facilitates decision regarding use of immunosuppression in patient with high activity score whereas in patient with only high chronicity index the immunosuppression needs to be reduced and plan for renal preservation needs to be made (Table 7.4).

Table 7.4: Activity and chronicity index			
Activity index		*Chronicity index*	
Endocapilary hypercellularity	0–3	Total glomerulosclerosis score	0–3
Neutrophils/karyorrhexis	0–3	Fibrous crescents	0–3
Fibrinoid necrosis	(0–3) × 2	Tubular atrophy	0–3
Hyaline deposits	0–3	Interstitial fibrosis	0–3
Cellular/fibro-cellular crescents	(0–3) × 2		
Interstitial Inflammation	0–3		
TOTAL	**0–24**		**0–12**

*0–3 is based on % involvement.

MANAGEMENT OF LUPUS NEPHRITIS

The aim of management is to control symptoms and signs, control inflammation, reduce damage in the kidney with minimal drug toxicity.

Supportive Management

Ultraviolet light is a potent trigger for disease activity in SLE. In addition to cutaneous flares, UV-B exposure has been reported to precipitate systemic flares.[16] Patients need to be counselled regarding avoidance of UV-B light during peak hours from 10 AM to 4 PM. Sunscreens with sun protection factor (SPF) of at least 30 should be applied 30 minutes prior to any sun exposure.[17] In resource constrained situations like our country full sleeved clothes, use of an umbrella can provide good sun protection.

Effective control of hypertension using angiotensin converting enzyme inhibitors/ angiotensin receptor blockers (ACEi/ARBs) is paramount in reducing proteinuria due to glomerular hyperfiltration. Adequate dietary restriction of salt helps both in control of hypertension as well as reduction of edema. Diuretics are useful in reducing edema as well as in control of hypertension.

Patient counselling regarding need for long-term therapy, regular need for tests and follow-up, avoidance of conception during active disease, possible side effects of drugs goes a long way in ensuring compliance and better outcomes. In addition, various options available should be discussed with the patient and a shared decision should be made.

High-dose or low-dose cyclophosphamide (CP) based induction therapy or mycophenolate induction are various options. Low-dose Euro lupus treatment protocol has been shown to be effective in inducing remission in Caucasian populations with minimal effect on fertility. In high dose NIH regimen of CP, GnRH agonists like leuprolide (3.75 mg IM 2 weeks prior to the cyclophosphamide dosage) can be used to preserve fertility.[18] Effective counselling regarding the teratogenicity of mycophenolic acid as well as CP also need to be told to patient.

Drug Therapy

Class I and II LN are known to have excellent renal prognosis and are most commonly asymptomatic. Current recommendations do not advocate treatment for these lesions. Aggressive immunosuppression is required for patients with class III and IV lupus nephritis and these are the patients who often present with nephritic syndrome and rapidly deteriorating renal function. Class V lupus nephritis typically presents with nephrotic syndrome and may resemble idiopathic membranous nephropathy and generally has a more favorable prognosis than class III and IV. Of note, class V lesions may co-exist with class III and IV in the revised ISN/RPS classification, in which case therapy should be tailored to the more aggressive regimens required for proliferative phenotype of class III and IV (Fig. 7.2).

In 2019, European League of Association of Rheumatology (EULAR) has given treatment guidelines for lupus nephritis which are easy to practice (Table 7.5).[19] The recent recommendations have added calcineurin inhibitor class of drugs based on multiple studies mainly from Asian cohorts.

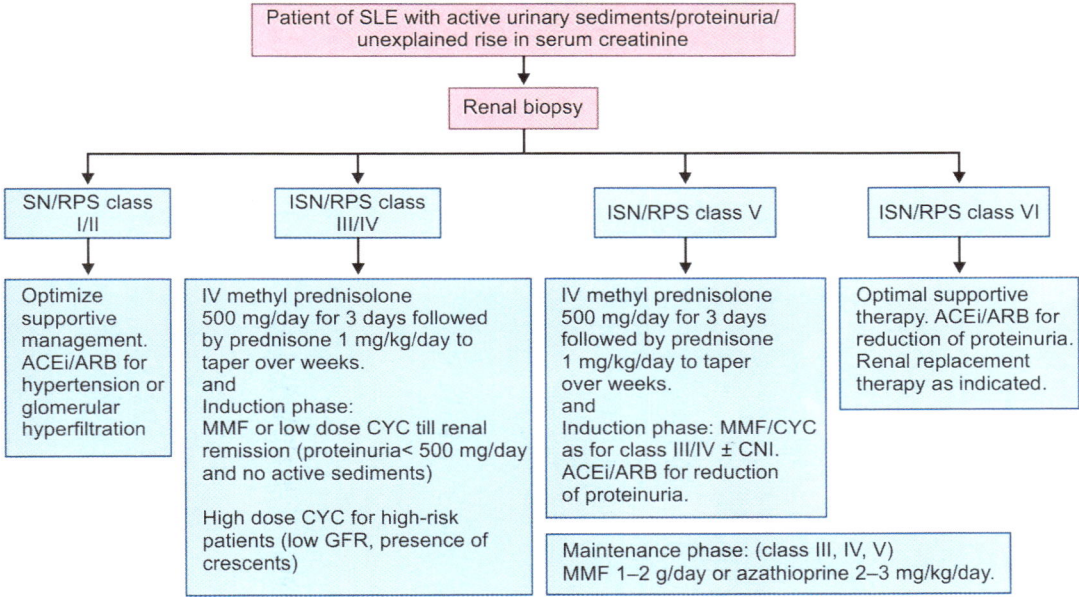

Fig. 7.2: A flow diagram showing the approach to a patient with suspected lupus nephritis

SPECIAL SITUATIONS

Lupus Podocytopathy

Patients with class I or II nephritis on biopsy who have an unexplained nephrotic range proteinuria may in fact have lupus podocytopathy that can only be diagnosed on electron microscopy. These patients generally respond to 1 mg/kg prednisone equivalent and form a unique group which requires treatment despite not having proliferative changes on biopsy.[13] Tacrolimus may also be useful in podocytopathy due to its ability to cause contraction of the effaced foot processes that are pathognomonic of lupus podocytopathy.

Case 3: A 24-year-old lady was diagnosed with SLE in 2006 when she presented with oral ulcers, fever and mild thrombocytopenia. She was treated with low dose prednisolone and hydroxy chloroquine. She was found to have anti-Ro and moderate levels of anti-cardiolipin antibodies. The patient subsequently had one pregnancy terminating in still birth at 30 weeks despite use of low-dose aspirin. In 2010, she was noticed to

Table 7.5: EULAR recommendations for management of lupus nephritis 2019

Recommendation (level/strength of recommendation)	Remark
Early recognition of signs of renal involvement and when present performance of a diagnostic renal biopsy are essential to ensure optimal outcomes **(2b/B)**.	
Mycophenolate **(1a/A)** or low-dose intravenous cyclophosphamide **(2a/B)** are recommended as initial (induction) treatment, as they have the best efficacy/toxicity ratio.	MMF: 2–3 grams/day. CYC: 500 mg IV every 15 days for 6 doses.
In patients at high risk for renal failure (reduced glomerular filtration rate, histological presence of fibrous crescents or fibrinoid necrosis, or tubular atrophy/interstitial fibrosis), similar regimens may be considered but high-dose intravenous cyclophosphamide can also be used **(1b/A)**.	CYC: 750 mg/m^2 body surface area every month for 7 doses. Increased CYC dose by 25% for every subsequent dose targeting a TLC nadir of 3000/mm^3.
For maintenance therapy, mycophenolate **(1a/A)** or azathioprine **(1a/A)** should be used. In cases with stable/improved renal function but incomplete renal response (persistent proteinuria >0.8–1 g/24 hours after at least 1 year of immunosuppressive treatment), repeat biopsy can distinguish chronic from active kidney lesions **(4/C)**.	MMF: 1–2 grams/day AZA: 2–3 mg/kg/day
Mycophenolate may be combined with low dose of a calcineurin inhibitor in severe nephrotic syndrome **(2b/C)** or incomplete renal response **(4/C)**, in the absence of uncontrolled hypertension, high chronicity index at kidney biopsy and/or reduced GFR.	Tacrolimus 0.1 mg/kg/day up titrated to the trough tacrolimus level of 4–6 ng/ml 12 hours after last dose of tacrolimus.

have hypertension and serum creatinine elevation to 2.1 mg/dl. Her urine showed bland sediment and proteinuria of 2.6 g/24 hours. A renal biopsy showed glomerular sclerosis, focal cortical atrophy and fibrous intimal hyperplasia of vessel wall. A diagnosis of chronic APS nephropathy was made.

APS Nephropathy

Antiphospholipid (APL) antibodies are associated with a worse renal prognosis in patients with lupus nephritis and have been associated with higher rates of chronic renal insufficiency. These antibodies are seen more commonly in biopsy proven membranous lupus nephritis.[20] APS nephropathy is characterized by features of a thrombotic microangiopathy on biopsy with interlobular fibrous intimal hyperplasia, arterial and arteriolar recanalizing thrombi, fibrous arterial occlusion, and focal cortical atrophy.[21] Clinical manifestations may include hypertension, proteinuria ranging from minimal to nephrotic level, hematuria and features of renal insufficiency.

There is no current consensus on the management of APS nephropathy due to lack of good prospective data. Patients who meet standard diagnostic criteria for APS should receive therapeutic anticoagulation as per norm.[22] Coexisting lupus nephritis warrants the use of hydroxychloroquine and standard immunosuppressive regimen.[23] Hypertension and proteinuria should be managed with ACEi/ARBs.

Refractory Lupus Nephritis

Any patient with persistent renal activity even after 6–12 months after induction therapy can be labeled as refractory lupus nephritis. Four weekly doses of rituximab (375 mg/m^2)

along with cyclophosphamide (500 mg/m^2) administered in 2 doses 3 weeks apart has been shown to improve overall renal function and reduce proteinuria in patients with refractory lupus nephritis.[24] However, a randomized control trial that evaluated addition of rituximab to standard of care including MMF and steroids did not show any additional benefit. Still RTX is used in patients with refractory LN with good success.

DURATION OF THERAPY

There is no consensus on how long to give maintenance therapy but most would prefer to give it for a minimum of 3 years and preferably for 5 years. Regular follow-up for early flare detection, control of hypertension, drug compliance and drug toxicity needs to be done 3–6 monthly. Regular use of hydroxychloroquine has been shown to reduce the incidence of relapse so it should be continued even after stopping maintenance therapy.

OUTCOME

The health-related quality of life is not significantly lower in lupus nephritis patients compared with SLE patients without lupus nephritis.[4] The overall survival rates of patients with lupus nephritis has steadily improved over the last 2 decades.[25] The cumulative incidence of death in LN at 10 years post diagnosis was 5.9% in the SLICC cohort (95% CI: 3.3% to 8.4%).[4] In the SLICC network, the cumulative incidence of end-stage renal disease among all patients of SLE was 4.6% and the cumulative incidence of ESRD in lupus nephritis patients was 10.1%.[4] ISN/RPS class IV lupus nephritis was associated with development of ESRD with a hazard ratio of 2.99 (95% CI 1.04 to 8.62) as compared to other classes.[4]

The outcomes are not as good in resource poor countries. In a study on 188 patients with LN from India survival with normal renal function at 5, 10, and 15 years was 84%, 69%, and 57%.[26] Another study with 134 children with LN showed actuarial ESRD-free survival at 5, 10 and 15 years of 91.1%, 79% and 76.2%, and 5, 10- and 15-year renal survival of 93.8%, 87.1% and 84%, respectively.[27] The main cause of death are cardiorespiratory illness and infections. In India, tuberculosis is also an important contributor to mortality and morbidity.[26,27]

Renal replacement therapy with transplantation has good success rate with 10–12% graft failure rate at 10 years. The recurrence rate for LN in grafted kidney is also low. The overall survival and graft survival is no different than transplantation for other causes.[28]

In conclusion, LN outcome has improved over last decades due to early diagnosis, use of immunosuppressive drugs, prolonged maintenance therapy and regular follow-up. Still we have a long way to go as a significant proportion of patient still develop ESRD and require renal replacement therapy.

REFERENCES

1. Wang H, Ren Y, Chang J, Gu L, Sun L-Y. A systematic review and meta-analysis of prevalence of biopsy-proven lupus nephritis. Arch Rheumatol. 2017 Jul 25;33(1):17–25.
2. Yap DYH, Chan TM. Lupus nephritis in Asia: Clinical features and management. Kidney Dis. 2015 Sep;1(2):100–9.
3. Almaani S, Meara A, Rovin BH. Update on lupus nephritis. Clin J Am Soc Nephrol. 2017 May 8; 12(5):825–35.
4. Hanly JG, O'Keeffe AG, Su L, Urowitz MB, Romero-Diaz J, Gordon C, et al. The frequency and outcome of lupus nephritis: results from an international inception cohort study. Rheumatology. 2016 Feb;55(2):252–62.

5. Haadlj E, Cervera R. Do we still need renal biopsy in lupus nephritis? Reumatologia. 2016;54(2):61–6.

6. Barancwska-Daca E, Choi YJ, Barrios R, Nassar G, Suki WN, Truong LD. Nonlupus nephritides in patients with systemic lupus erythematosus: A comprehensive clinicopathologic study and review of the literature. Hum Pathol. 2001 Oct;32(10):1125–35.

7. Shea-Simonds P, Cairns TD, Roufosse C, Cook T, Vyse TJ. Lupus podocytopathy. Rheumatology. 2009 Dec 1;48(12):1616–8.

8. Bomback AS, Markowitz GS. Lupus podocytopathy: A distinct entity. Clin J Am Soc Nephrol CJASN. 2016 Apr 7;11(4):547–8.

9. Hahn BH, McMahon M, Wilkinson A, Wallace WD, Daikh DI, FitzGerald J, et al. American College of Rheumatology Guidelines for Screening, Case Definition, Treatment and Management of Lupus Nephritis. Arthritis Care Res. 2012 Jun;64(6):797–808.

10. Bertsias GK, Tektonidou M, Amoura Z, Aringer M, Bajema I, Berden JHM, et al. Joint European League Against Rheumatism and European Renal Association-European Dialysis and Transplant Association (EULAR/ERA-EDTA) recommendations for the management of adult and paediatric lupus nephritis. Ann Rheum Dis. 2012 Nov;71(11):1771–82.

11. McRae M, Rousseau-Gagnon M, Philibert D, Houde I, Riopel J, Latulippe E, et al. The interpretation of repeat renal biopsies in patients with lupus nephritis. Rheumatol Oxf Engl. 2014 Jun;53(6):1151–2.

12. Narváez J, Ricse M, Gomà M, Mitjavila F, Fulladosa X, Capdevila O, et al. The value of repeat biopsy in lupus nephritis flares. Medicine (Baltimore). 2017 Jun;96(24):e7099.

13. Hu W, Chen Y, Wang S, Chen H, Liu Z, Zeng C, et al. Clinical-morphological features and outcomes of lupus podocytopathy. Clin J Am Soc Nephrol CJASN. 2016 Apr 7;11(4):585–92.

14. Bajema IM, Wilhelmus S, Alpers CE, Bruijn JA, Colvin RB, Haas M, et al. Revision of the International Society of Nephrology/Renal Pathology Society classification for lupus nephritis: Clarification of definitions, and modified National Institutes of Health activity and chronicity indices. Kidney Int. 2018 Apr;93(4):789–796.

15. Austin HA, Muenz LR, Joyce KM, Antonovych TT, Balow JE. Diffuse proliferative lupus nephritis: Identification of specific pathologic features affecting renal outcome. Kidney Int. 1984 Apr;25(4):689–95.

16. Schmidt E, Tony H-P, Brocker E-B, Kneitz C. Sun-induced life-threatening lupus nephritis. Ann N Y Acad Sci. 2007 Jun 1;1108(1):35–40.

17. Kuhn A, Gensch K, Haust M, Meuth A-M, Boyer F, Dupuy P, et al. Photoprotective effects of a broad-spectrum sunscreen in ultraviolet-induced cutaneous lupus erythematosus: a randomized, vehicle-controlled, double-blind study. J Am Acad Dermatol. 2011 Jan;64(1):37–48.

18. Somers EC, Marder W, Christman GM, Ognenovski V, McCune WJ. Use of a gonadotropin-releasing hormone analog for protection against premature ovarian failure during cyclophosphamide therapy in women with severe lupus. Arthritis Rheum. 2005 Sep;52(9):2761–7.

19. Fanouriakis A, Kostopoulou M, Alunno A, Aringer M, Bajema I, Boletis JN, et al. 2019 update of the EULAR recommendations for the management of systemic lupus erythematosus. Ann Rheum Dis. 2019 Jun 1;78(6):736–45.

20. Moroni G, Ventura D, Riva P, Panzeri P, Quaglini S, Banfi G, et al. Antiphospholipid antibodies are associated with an increased risk for chronic renal insufficiency in patients with lupus nephritis. Am J Kidney Dis Off J Natl Kidney Found. 2004 Jan;43(1):28–36.

21. Nochy D, Daugas E, Droz D, Beaufils H, Grünfeld JP, Piette JC, et al. The intrarenal vascular lesions associated with primary antiphospholipid syndrome. J Am Soc Nephrol JASN. 1999 Mar;10(3):507–18.

22. Tektonidou MG. Antiphospholipid syndrome nephropathy: From pathogenesis to treatment. Front Immunol. 2018 May 31;9:1181.

23. Tektonidou MG. Identification and treatment of APS renal involvement. Lupus. 2014 Oct;23(12):1276–8.

24. Kronbichler A, Brezina B, Gauckler P, Quintana LF, Jayne DRW. Refractory lupus nephritis: When, why and how to treat. Autoimmun Rev. 2019;18(5):510–18.

25. Bernatsky S, Boivin J-F, Joseph L, Manzi S, Ginzler E, Gladman DD, et al. Mortality in systemic lupus erythematosus. Arthritis Rheum. 2006 Aug;54(8):2550–7.

26. Dhir V, Aggarwal A, Lawrence A, Agarwal V, Misra R. Long term outcome of lupus nephritis in Asian Indians. Arthritis Care Res (Hoboken). 2012; 64:713–20.
27. Srivastava P, Abujam B, Misra R, Lawrence A, Agarwal V, Aggarwal A. Outcome of lupus nephritis in childhood onset SLE in North and central India: Single centre experience over 25 years. Lupus 2016;25:1–11.
28. Kim JE, Kim YC, Min SL, Lee H, Ha J, Chin HJ, Kim YS, Han SS. Transplant outcomes in kidney recipients with lupus nephritis, and systematic review. Lupus. 2020 Mar;29(3):248–55.

Abdominal Pain: Physicians Nightmare

Abhishek Zanwar, Ramnath Misra

INTRODUCTION

Gastrointestinal involvement is common in SLE with nearly 40% of lupus patients experiencing some form of gastrointestinal symptoms in the course of their disease.[1] Abdominal pain in a patient with lupus can be due to various causes, ranging from drug intolerance to serious causes like enteritis, pancreatitis, mesenteric vasculitis or vaso-occlusive disease. Assessment of global disease activity, review of drugs are important considerations while assessing a patient with abdominal pain. In this review article we will be illustrating how to approach and manage case of lupus with abdominal pain.

Case 1: A 28-year-old married lady with 2 children was diagnosed anti-phospholipid antibody syndrome 3 years ago when she had digital gangrene. She was treated with aspirin and HCQ until 2 months when she stopped both the drgus due to epistaxis. Now, she presented with epigastric pain, constipation and recurrent vomiting of 15 days duration. There was no melena. She had history of 3 recurrent abortions. On examination she was locking sick but was conscious and co-operative. There was bilateral vesicular breath sound with crepitations. She had loud P2 however there was no murmur. Abdomen was soft, mildly tender and bowel sounds were absent. There was no hepatosplenomegaly or free fluid. Ultrasound of abdomen showed gall stones with ascites. While X-ray of abdomen in erect posture showed multiple air-fluid level (Fig. 8.1). With possibility of mesenteric ischemia, CT abdomen with triple phase was done which showed multifocal enhancing mural thickening in small bowel loops with mucosal enhancement, edematous colonic wall, with few areas of small bowel luminal narrowing. All vessels were normal. Mesenteric vascular engorgement was seen with typical Coombs' and target sign (Fig. 8.2a and b). ANA was positive and she also had raised anti-dsDNA antibodies and low complement levels. A diagnosis of SLE, with secondary APS and mesenteric vasculitis was made and she was treated with high dose pulse steroid followed by cyclophosphamide and prednisolone. Anticoagulation was also started with which she gradually improved.

APPROACH TO CASE OF LUPUS WITH ABDOMINAL PAIN

A detailed history is of paramount importance in approaching a lupus patient with abdominal pain to identify sinister causes from minor or less important causes. Patients with SLE can have disease-related or unrelated causes of abdominal pain (Table 8.1), many of these could be serious manifestation of disease itself. As patients are usually on

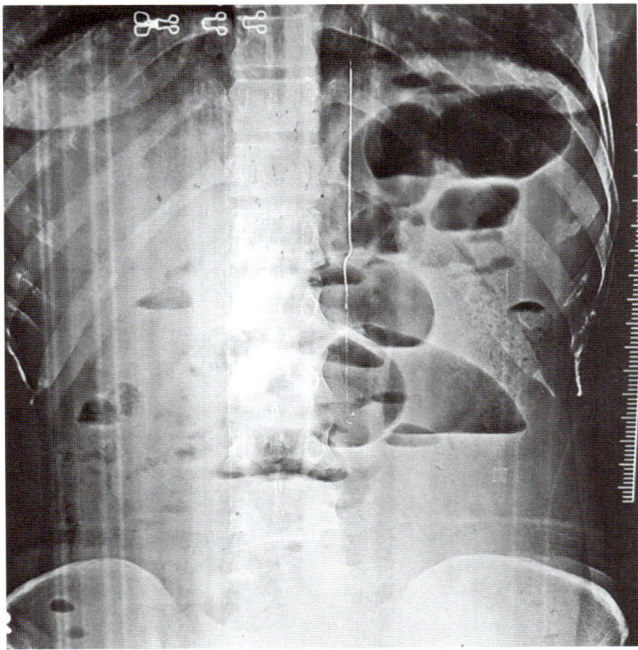

Fig. 8.1: Dilated bowel loops with multiple air–fluid levels in case of lupus enteritis

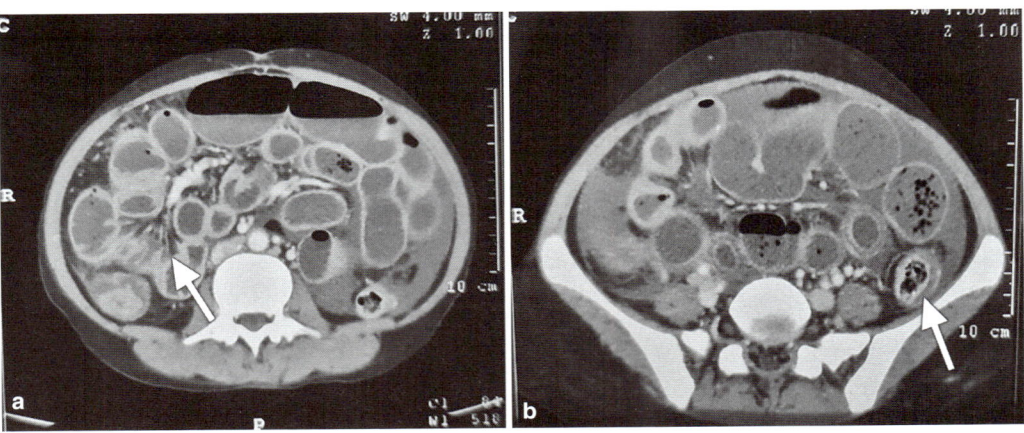

Fig. 8.2a and b: CT showing: **(a)** Coombs' and **(b)** target sign (double halo) marked by arrowhead in case 1 suggestive of lupus enteritis

immunosuppressive (IS) treatment, typical clinical features may be absent at the time of presentation.

Red flag features signifying serious causes are sudden onset of pain, continuous pain, associated vomiting and hypotension, gastrointestinal bleeding, guarding or rigidity of abdomen. Such patients need adequate resuscitative measures and institution of empirical management of suspected cause till diagnosis is clear. If patients has clinically active SLE

Table 8.1: Etiology of abdominal pain in case of SLE

Lupus related	Unrelated
Peritonitis	Gastrointestinal/urinary tract infection
Lupus enteritis	Peptic ulcer disease, perforation
Pancreatitis	Drug-induced gastritis
Mesenteric vasculitis/thrombosis	Adrenal insufficiency
Intestinal pseudo-obstruction	Atherosclerosis of abdominal aorta
Veno-occlusive disease	Nephrolithiasis
Lupus hepatitis	Irritable bowel syndrome

then lupus related etiologies like lupus enteritis, pancreatitis, mesenteric vasculitis and thrombosis and rarely intestinal pseudo-obstruction needs to be considered. In contrast, in patients on high dose of IS drugs with well controlled lupus activity, causes like gastrointestinal infection, peptic ulcer disease, and intestinal perforation should be suspected.

Though global disease activity remains a good guide for initial evaluation, sometimes picture may not be as clear, since isolated SLE-related gastrointestinal manifestations are not uncommon and patient with active systemic disease can develop gastrointestinal infections due to ongoing IS treatment. Patients without red flag features usually have either milder manifestation of lupus like peritonitis or common causes like drug-induced gastritis.

Detailed history of pain like; onset of pain, nature (colicky, dull aching, sharp, burning, etc.), location, radiation to other site, associated vomiting or diarrhea, aggravating and relieving factors can help in the determination of a probable diagnosis. Location of abdominal pain is important to narrow down differential diagnosis (Table 8.2). Onset and duration of pain can also help. Pancreatitis, an important cause of pain abdomen usually causes insidious onset of persistent pain, which may increase in severity gradually. Pain due to peritonitis is usually acute onset and reaches to maximum intensity quickly. Other lupus-related pathologies, which have acute onset pain are, lupus enteritis, veno-occlusive disease. Nature

Table 8.2: Location of pain and probable pathology

Right upper quadrant	Epigastric region	Left upper quadrant
Budd-Chiari syndrome	Pancreatitis	Splenomegaly
Portal vein thrombosis	Peptic ulcer disease	Splenic infarct
Lupus hepatitis	Drug-induced gastritis	
Cholecystitis	Functional dyspepsia	
Lower abdominal pain	Lupus enteritis	
Atherosclerosis of abdominal aorta		
Pyelonephritis		
Infective enteritis/colitis		

Diffuse abdominal pain

Peritonitis
Mesenteric vasculitis/thrombosis
Intestinal pseudo-obstruction
Gastrointestinal perforation
Adrenal insufficiency
Irritable bowel syndrome

of abdominal pain is important clue for origin of pain. Colicky pain is usually related to hollow visceral structure pathology like, intestinal pseudo-obstruction or ureteric stone. Dull aching pain is related to other structures like liver, pancreas. Burning pain is usually due to gastritis or gastro-esophageal reflux. Sharp pain can be due to acute veno-occlusive disease or a splenic infarct. Radiation to other sites is quite characteristic for certain etiologies. Pain of pancreatitis usually refers to back while that due to urolithiasis refers to groin. Radiation to shoulder or inter-scapular area can be due to sub-diaphragmatic pathologies like cholecystitis or cholelitiasis. Aggravation of abdominal pain with food is usually seen with a vascular pathology (mesenteric vasculitis/thrombosis, atherosclerosis of abdominal aorta) or chronic pancreatic insufficiency. As against pain due to peptic ulcer disease of duodenum will be relieved with food. Pain of pancreatitis is less intense on leaning forward or sitting.

History of associated symptoms especially vomiting, containing bile along with constipation suggests intestinal obstruction. Melena can be associated with peptic ulcer or lupus enteritis. Infective colitis can cause hematochezia. Burning micturition, oliguria/anuria and high grade spiking fever point towards urosepsis.

Importance of reviewing drugs taken by patient cannot be overemphasized. Non-steroidal anti-inflammatory drugs (NSAID), steroids can cause gastritis and peptic ulcer disease. Immunosuppressive agent like mycophenolate mofetil (MMF) is more likely to cause gastrointestinal upset.[2] High-dose steroid has been implicated to be a cause for pancreatitis but distinction between disease-related and steroid-induced pancreatitis is difficult, especially in the setting where pulse doses of steroids are used. There have been multiple case reports of azathioprine (AZA) and MMF-induced pancreatitis.[3,4] Patients undergoing induction therapy for lupus nephritis can develop gastrointestinal infection due to combination of high-dose steroids and cyclophosphamide (CYC)/rituximab (RTX)/MMF.

CLINICAL MANIFESTATION

Some patients can have hypothalmopituitary axis suppression due to long-term use of steroids and may present with nausea, abdominal pain and vomiting due to adrenal insufficiency. Specific gastrointestinal manifestations of lupus presenting as abdominal pain are described below.

Lupus Enteritis

Lupus enteritis is a form of vasculitis usually involving small bowel. It is included in the British Isles Lupus Assessment Group (BILAG) disease activity index.[5] Patients commonly present with abdominal pain, worsening after food intake which may be accompanied by ascites, vomiting or diarrhea.[6] Diagnosis is supported by either imaging or biopsy. Overall prevalence of up to 6% has been reported.[6] Females are affected more frequently (85%) with median age of onset pf 34 years. Though isolated lupus enteritis has been reported, it is uncommon and is usually associated with active disease involving other organs in one third of cases.[7] It is characterized by bowel wall thickening, dilatation of bowel loops (Fig. 8.2) and 'target sign' on computed tomogram (Fig. 8.3).[8] It should be noted that target sign or hallow sign is not specific for lupus enteritis and can be seen in various other disorders including infective colitis.[9]

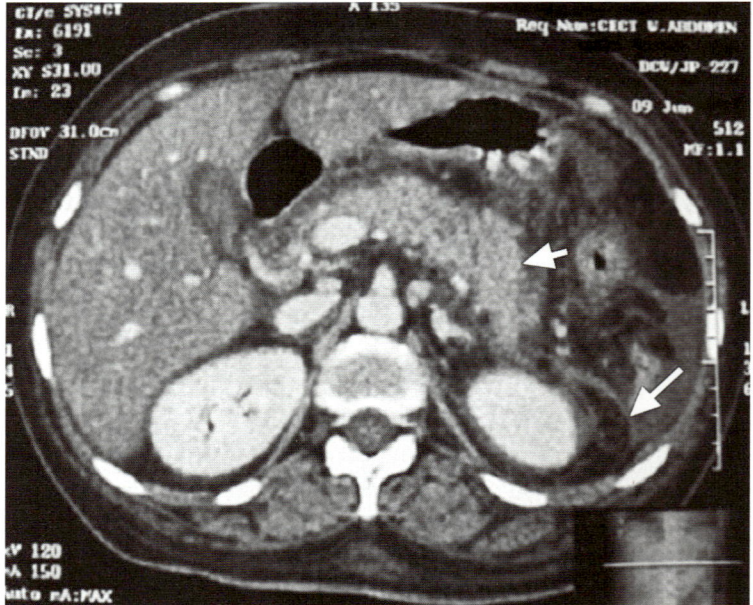

Fig. 8.3: Bulky pancreas with fat stranding in case 2 suggestive of acute pancreatitis

Lupus Peritonitis

Though estimated prevalence is 10%, autopsy studies have shown higher prevalence of up to 60% of cases.[10] Again isolated peritonitis is rare but can develop in early phase of flare. Usually it responds to treatment but in some cases it can become chronic and may lead to peritoneal thickening and adhesions.

Case 2: A 9-years-old girl was admitted with acute abdominal pain for 2 days. She had history of fever and malar rash for last 2 months and the fever had become persistent since last 2 weeks. 2 days ago, she started having abdominal pain, which was sudden in onset, was present all over abdomen but was more prominent at epigastric area and was associated with vomiting of non-bilious content. Pain was lessened by sitting up was aggravated by lying down. She had malar rash and joint pain. With suspicion of acute pancreatitis serum amylase and lipase levels ordered and was found to be increased 3–4 times the upper limit. Imaging with computed tomogram (CT) scan (Fig. 8.3) confirmed diagnosis of acute pancreatitis. There was no evidence of mesenteric vasculitis or enteritis. Her anti-nuclear antibody was positive and serum anti-dsDNA levels were raised. She also had proteinuria with active urinary sediments. She was treated with pulse methylprednisolone doses and followed by cyclophosphamide. She achieved remission by the end of 3 months.

Lupus-associated Pancreatitis

The prevalence is reported up to 4%.[11] Pancreatitis usually occurs in early phase of disease and in 22% it can be present at the time of presentation. In a retrospective cohort of 71 lupus pancreatitis cases, hypertriglyceridemia, psychosis and pleurisy were associated with risk of pancreatitis attributable to lupus.[12] In the same study, anti-La antibody was associated with pancreatitis while anti-phospholipid antibodies were not. Though pancreatitis in the setting of lupus is usually acute, rare cases of chronic pancreatitis have been reported.[13]

Mesenteric Vasculitis or Thrombosis

Although rare, mesenteric vasculitis is a serious manifestation of lupus. Patient usually has anorexia, abdominal pain on intake of food sometimes associated with vomiting, diarrhea and weight loss, especially if it's chronic. If unrecognized for long it can lead to perforation due to intestinal infarction. Like lupus enteritis this entity can also be associated with anti-phospholipid syndrome.[14]

Intestinal Pseudo-obstruction

Like mesenteric vasculitis this is also rare and can rarely be the presenting manifestation of lupus. Usually presents with classic signs and symptoms of bowel obstruction. The obstruction is not anatomical, hence the term pseudo-obstruction. It is considered to be immune-mediated dysfunction of the smooth muscles of the bowel leading to hypomotility.[15]

Lupus Hepatitis

Usually it presents with insidious onset of anorexia, fatigue. When severe, it causes hepatomegaly, abdominal pain and jaundice. Liver enzymes are mildly raised but higher levels can be found in severe cases. Although frequent associations with anti-ribosomal P antibody have been described, a direct pathogenic role has not been proven.[16] Liver biopsy demonstrates peri-portal lymphocytic infiltrates with isolated areas of necrosis.

INVESTIGATIONS

Imaging is immensely helpful in ruling out serious pathologies. Plain X-ray of abdomen can give the first clue for perforation or intestinal obstruction. Ultrasonography (USG) of abdomen usually shows bowel wall edema in patients with enteritis. Though USG can detect evidence of pancreatitis, it is less sensitive than CT scan. Doppler evaluation can reveal the presence of hepatic veno-occlusive disease. CT scan can be diagnostic for etiologies like pancreatitis, mesenteric vasculitis/thrombosis. CT scan is not only useful for the diagnosis of pancreatitis but also for the evaluation of severity and complications associated with it like necrosis, pseudocyst formation and detection of arterial aneurysm. 'Double halo' or 'Target sign' (Fig. 8.3) though typically seen in most cases of lupus enteritis is not specific and can be seen in other conditions like infective etiologies and ischemia also. Another feature of mesenteric vasculitis is presence of Comb sign which can be seen in up to 70% of cases.[7] Congestion and engorgement of mesenteric vessels gives rise to comb like appearance. In addition, mesenteric attenuation can be seen in cases of mesenteric vasculitis. Apart from vasculitic manifestations CT scan can also detect thrombotic manifestation like veno-occlusive disease and splenic infarct.

Apart from imaging, biochemical parameters are useful for the diagnosis of pancreatitis or hepatitis. Serum amylase and lipase levels more than three times the upper limit of normal suggest acute pancreatitis, while those of serum glutamic oxaloacetic transaminase (SGOT) and serum glutamic pyruvic transaminase (SGPT) suggest hepatitis. Though sensitive, biochemical parameters are not specific.

Evaluation of systemic disease activity is important. Serum anti-dsDNA titers, complement levels help in determination of global disease activity. As gastrointestinal manifestations are associated with other internal organ involvement like nephritis, screening tests and detailed evaluation should be done accordingly.

Peritoneal fluid examination should be done especially in absence of systemic disease activity. Infections like tuberculosis need to be excluded before making a diagnosis of isolated lupus peritonitis. Ascitic fluid adenosine deaminase levels, especially in high titers suggests tuberculosis.

Lupus unrelated etiologies like urinary tract infections, urolithiasis or cholecystitis could be diagnosed on imaging. CT scan is more sensitive than USG for evaluation. Specific investigation like urine culture also needs to be done in clinically relevant setting. An algorithmic approach for abdominal pain in patients with SLE is illustrated in Fig. 8.4.

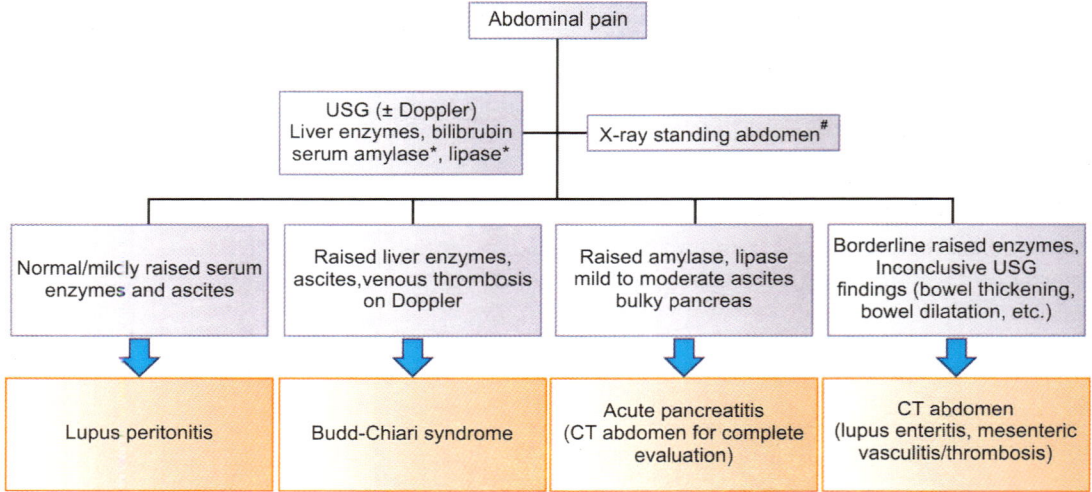

*If suspected pancreatitis, # if suspected intestinal obstruction/pseudo-obstruction
CT—computed tomogram; USG—ultra-sonogram

Fig. 8.4: An algorithmic approach for abdominal pain patient with SLE

TREATMENT

Treatment is usually guided by the diagnosis and its severity. Vasculitic manifestation like enteritis, pancreatitis or mesenteric vasculitis is usually treated with high-dose steroids and upfront use of immunosuppressive agents like cyclophosphamide or MMF.[7] Milder manifestations like peritonitis can be managed with prednisolone and either methotrexate or azathioprine. Lupus hepatitis is usually treated with steroids and azathioprine or MMF.

Anti-coagulation is usually initiated for cases of veno-occlusive disease unless contraindicated due to high bleeding risk. Whenever temporal association with drug and adverse event is strong, the suspected drug needs to be stopped especially with etiologies like pancreatitis.

Surgical interventions may be needed in case of intestinal pseudo-obstruction when conservative management with steroids and immunosuppressive agent fails. Perforation and gangrene of bowel are other situations when surgical management is needed.

To summarize, abdominal pain in lupus can be due to either disease-related or unrelated causes. Based on clinical features, stratifying patients according to suspected etiology can help in early recognition of pathology. Global disease activity and drug history are important clues. Imaging using X-ray, US and CT are crucial for correct diagnosis. Specific management should be initiated at the earliest and if required surgical intervention should be sought early.

REFERENCES

1. Sultan SM, Ioannou Y, Isenberg DA. A review of gastrointestinal manifestations of systemic lupus erythematosus. Rheumatol Oxf Engl. 1999 Oct;38(10):917–32.
2. Zwerner J, Fiorentino D. Mycophenolate mofetil. Dermatol Ther. 2007 Jul–Aug;20(4):229–38.
3. Einollahi B, Dolatimehr F. Acute pancreatitis induced by mycophenolate mofetil in a kidney transplant patient. J Nephropharmacology. 2015 Feb 18;4(2):72–4.
4. Teich N, Mohl W, Bokemeyer B, Bündgens B, Büning J, Miehlke S, et al. Azathioprine-induced acute pancreatitis in patients with inflammatory bowel diseases—a prospective study on incidence and severity. J Crohns Colitis. 2016 Jan;10(1):61–8.
5. Isenberg DA, Rahman A, Allen E, Farewell V, Akil M, Bruce IN, et al. BILAG 2004. Development and initial validation of an updated version of the British Isles Lupus Assessment Group's disease activity index for patients with systemic lupus erythematosus. Rheumatology. 2005 Jul 1;44(7):902–6.
6. Koo BS, Hong S, Kim YJ, Kim Y-G, Lee C-K, Yoo B. Lupus enteritis: Clinical characteristics and predictive factors for recurrence. Lupus. 2015 May;24(6):628–32.
7. Janssens P, Arnaud L, Galicier L, Mathian A, Hie M, Sene D, et al. Lupus enteritis: From clinical findings to therapeutic management. Orphanet J Rare Dis. 2013 May 3;8:67.
8. Patro PS, Phatak S, Zanwar A, Lawrence A. Presumptive lupus enteritis. Am J Med. 2016 Nov; 129(11):e277–8.
9. Ahualli J. The target sign: Bowel wall. Radiology. 2005 Feb;234(2):549–50.
10. Takeno M, Ishigatsubo Y. Intestinal manifestations in systemic lupus erythematosus. Intern Med Tokyo Jpn. 2006;45(2):41–2.
11. Pascual-Ramos V, Duarte-Rojo A, Villa AR, Hernández-Cruz B, Alarcón-Segovia D, Alcocer-Varela J, et al. Systemic lupus erythematosus as a cause and prognostic factor of acute pancreatitis. J Rheumatol. 2004 Apr;31(4):707–12.
12. Makol A, Petri M. Pancreatitis in systemic lupus erythematosus: Frequency and associated factors—a review of the Hopkins Lupus Cohort. J Rheumatol. 2010 Feb;37(2):341–5.
13. Gutierrez SC, Pasqua AV, Casas H, Cremaschi MB, Valenzuela ML, Cubilla AA, et al. Chronic pancreatitis and systemic lupus erythematosus: An uncommon association. Case Rep Gastroenterol. 2008 Jan 10;2(1):6–10.
14. Cervera R, Espinosa G, Cordero A, Oltra MR, Unzurrunzaga A, Rossiñol T, et al. Intestinal involvement secondary to the antiphospholipid syndrome (APS): Clinical and immunologic characteristics of 97 patients: Comparison of classic and catastrophic APS. Semin Arthritis Rheum. 2007 Apr;36(5):287–96.
15. Mok MY, Wong RW, Lau CS. Intestinal pseudo-obstruction in systemic lupus erythematosus: an uncommon but important clinical manifestation. Lupus. 2000;9(1):11–8.
16. Ohira H, Takiguchi J, Rai T, Abe K, Yokokawa J, Sato Y, et al. High frequency of anti-ribosomal P antibody in patients with systemic lupus erythematosus-associated hepatitis. Hepatol Res Off J Jpn Soc Hepatol. 2004 Mar;28(3):137–9.

Neuropsychiatric Lupus: As Confusing as Ever

Vineeta Shobha, Benzeeta Pinto

INTRODUCTION

The clinical heterogeneity and complexity of lupus is best exemplified in neuropsychiatric manifestations of lupus (NPSLE). Almost all structures of central and peripheral nervous system may be affected. As there is no gold standard for diagnosis, a high index of clinical suspicion is necessary, alongside neuroimaging and laboratory findings, to establish diagnosis and to exclude other differentials.

It is well established that as many as 50% of lupus patients have neurological involvement during the course of their disease. Approximately, 40% of neuropsychiatric SLE (NPSLE) cases are a consequence of the disease process itself, where it is considered as primary, others being infections, metabolic disorders, and side effects of drugs.[1] We review the major NPSLE manifestations and discuss their clinical features, pathogenic mechanisms, radiological findings, and treatment options.

Case Vignette 1: A 25-year-old lady presents with athralgias and malar rash to her physician. Evaluation reveals WEC count of 3000 m³, rest of the blood counts are within normal limits. ANA, anti-DSDNA are positive with low complements and she is started on low dose steroids and hydroxychloroquine. She presents after 8 weeks with fever and involuntary movements of bilateral upper limbs with darting tongue. Patient is treated with haloperidol outside with some improvement. MRI reveals bilateral basal ganglia T2/FLAIR hyperintensities with no diffusion restriction (Fig. 9.1). MR angiogram is normal. ASLO titres are normal. She has leucopenia, thrombocytopenia with platelet count of 20,000 with low complements. Lupus anticoagulant is positive.

Haloperidol is continued and she is started on prednisolone 1 mg/kg body weight. She is started on azathioprine 2 mg/kg body weight. Her chorea gradually improves over the next 2 weeks. She is started on ecospirin and HCQ is continued. Steroids are gradually tapered over next 2 months. There is no recurrence of chorea.

The CNS manifestation in this patient is immune-mediated/inflammatory and associated with non CNS activity. Hence, this patient is treated with immunosuppression. The antiphospholipid antibodies are positive, however since no thrombosis is detected primary thromboprophylaxis with aspirin is given to this patient.

NPSLE SYNDROMES

In 1999, the ACR research committee, comprising experts from rheumatology, neurology, immunology, psychiatry and neuropsychology produced a standard nomenclature and set of case definitions for 19 NPSLE syndromes (Table 9.1).[2,3] These included the diagnostic criteria, important exclusion, and specific diagnostic tests (laboratory and imaging evaluation).[2,3] Prior to this, Kassan and Lokshin[4] had proposed one of the first classification criteria in 1979. How, et al.[5] subsequently classified neurologic manifestations of lupus as major and minor or focal and diffuse. These have been discussed in a recent review.[6] Although ACR classication includes syndromes with no clear pathophysiological mechanism and is not specific for neuropsychiatric events caused exclusively by SLE, it helps the physician recognize any neurological involvement. Risk factors associated with NPSLE include generalized SLE activity; previous neuropsychiatric events or other concurring neuropsychiatric manifestations; the presence of moderate to high titers of antiphospholipid antibodies (aPL) such as lupus anticoagulant and anticardiolipin or anti-β2 glycoprotein 1 (either IgG or IgM), especially in cerebrovascular disease, myelopathy, cognitive dysfunction, seizures and movement disorders; and anti-ribosomal P protein antibodies (anti-P antibodies), that have been associated with lupus psychosis in some studies.[7]

Headache occurs in up to 40% of SLE patients and may be associated with other NP events. However, the prevalence of two common types of headaches; tension-type headache, and migraine, does not differ between SLE and the general population.[8] Headache in SLE is not associated with a higher frequency of disease activity, and bio-markers such as aPL, anti-ribosomal P antibodies and other autoantibodies.[9] It is important to rule out other causes such as meningitis, cerebral venous sinus thrombosis, cerebral or subarachnoid hemorrhage and posterior reversible encephalopathy syndrome.[8]

Cognitive dysfunction may occur in 23–60% of lupus patients and is associated with aPL antibodies, steroid use, diabetes and low level of education.[10] Lupus anticoagulant positive

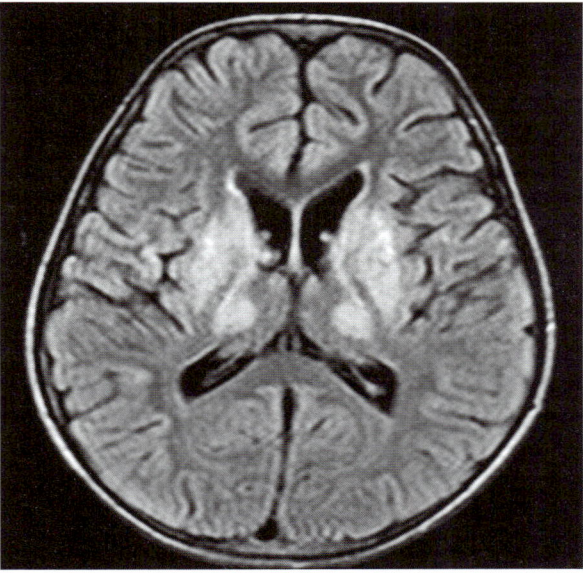

Fig. 9.1: MRI brain—T2 FLAIR sequence showing bilateral basal ganglia hyperintensities

Table 9.1: ACR case definitions of NPSLE

Central nervous system	Peripheral nervous system
Aseptic meningitis	Acute inflammatory demyelinating polyradiculoneuropathy
Acute confusional state	Autonomic disorders
Anxiety disorder	Cranial neuropathy
Cerebrovascular disease	Mononeuropathy
Cognitive dysfunction	Myasthenia gravis
Demyelinating syndrome	Plexopathy
Headache	Polyneuropathy
Movement disorder	
Mood disorders	
Myelopathy	
Psychosis	
Seizures	

lupus patients are three times more likely to have impaired neuropsychological functioning, with working memory dysfunction.[11] This is attributed to white matter changes and microvascular thrombosis. Depressive symptoms may also reduce cognitive function, but in lupus, cognitive dysfunction is not fully explained by depression alone. In a comparison of neuropsychological scores between patients with depression and those with depression and SLE, the latter showed even lower scores.[12]

Seizures occur in 12–22% of SLE patients and are associated with increased morbidity and mortality.[13,14] Seizures are associated with anti-phospholipid antibodies; disease activity, multiple NPSLE manifestations (e.g. psychosis, stroke) and severe baseline organ damage. Other risk factors for seizures include female sex and younger age. Inflammatory processes are believed to be a major player in the pathogenesis of seizures. Ischemic vascular disease and antibodies that bind to cerebral tissues such as anticardiolipin and anti-Sm have been associated with seizures. MRI of NPSLE patients with seizures show more gray matter hyper intensities and may develop brain atrophy.[15,16]

Acute confusional state is defined as disturbance in consciousness or alertness, and subsequent attention deficits that are accompanied by cognitive decline and/or affect or mood changes. Frequencies have varied in different cohorts from 0.9–8.0%.[17] It has been associated with the presence of anti-NR2/NMDAR antibodies and anti-Sm antibodies in the CSF. The etiopathogenic mechanism for acute confusional state in SLE is primarily inflammatory with increased production of inflammatory mediators, BBB disruption, and intrathecal immune complex formation. SLE patients with acute confusional state and high-intensity white matter lesions on MRI have greater mortality.[17,18]

Psychosis has been reported to occur in 3–12% of SLE patients from different cohorts.[19] Risk factor for psychosis include presence of anti-ribosomal-P antibodies in serum and CSF and serum antiendothelial antibodies.[7,19] It has shown that anti-ribosome P antibodies can bind to neuronal antigens, penetrate neuronal cells, and inhibit protein synthesis in neuronal cells and even induce neuronal apoptosis.[7] Clinically, glucocorticoid-induced psychosis must always be considered in the differential of lupus psychosis.

Mood disorders (anxiety and depression) occur in as many as 20% of SLE patients and are typically multifactorial.[20,21] A systematic review found a prevalence of 17% to 75% of depressive disorders among patients with SLE.[22] Mood disorders are associated with disease activity, high prednisone doses (≥20 mg), cutaneous disease and longitudinal extensive transverse myelitis. They may occur in isolation or in association with other NP manifestations and influences the quality of life negatively.[22] Neuroimaging or serological markers are not helpful for diagnosing mood and anxiety disorders, although anti-P and anti-NMDA receptor autoantibodies have been associated with a higher incidence of depression in patients with SLE.[21,22]

Cerebrovascular events (CVD) account for 10 to 15% of deaths in SLE patients.[23] Patients with SLE have a twofold increase in the risk of ischemic stroke, and a fourfold increase in the risk of sub-arachnoid hemorrhage compared to the general population.[24] Lupus disease severity, hypertension and hyperlipidemia are important predictors of stroke and stroke severity.[25] Accelerated atherosclerosis, and inflammatory mediators such as complement components, cytokines and aPL antibodies play key role in the development of CVD. Patients with SLE and stroke should be routinely screened for APS. A recent systematic review suggested fivefold increase in the risk of IS or transient ischemic attack in patients with aPL antibodies compared to controls.[26] Lupus anticoagulant is a stronger predictor of thrombosis amongst antiphospholipid antibodies. CNS vasculitis is a rare cause of stroke in SLE, accounting for 7% of cases in some case series.[24]

Movement disorders are uncommon neuropsychiatric manifestations in SLE. Chorea is the most described manifestation and may be the first manifestation in SLE occurring in 2% of adult patients, predominantly in women. It is believed to be related to aPL antibodies. Other movement disorders include parkinsonism, myoclonus and dystonias.[19]

Aseptic meningitis is reported in 1.4 to 1.6% in retrospective studies. Infective meningitis always needs exclusion.[27] Typically patients present with headache and altered mental status. Cerebrospinal fluid analysis may reveal lymphocytic cells and protein.

Lupus myelitis is reported in 1 to 1.5% of SLE patients. It may manifest as transverse myelitis or asymmetrical spinal cord syndrome, bladder involvement, neuropathic pain or presence of a sensory level. Ischemic/thrombotic myelopathy and or localized acute inflammation are postulated etio-pathologic mechanisms.[28] MRI studies reveal two distinct clinical patterns—gray-matter and white-matter myelitis. Patients with gray-matter myelitis often have a prodromal phase of fever and urinary retention at onset that rapidly evolves to paraplegia during disease activity. An MRI reveals spinal cord swelling and enhancement.[29] White-matter myelitis has been associated with a less severe presentation and slower progression. Neuromyelitis optica can also co-occur in SLE and are related to NMO-IgG anti-aquaporin 4 (AQP4) antibodies. NMO IgG is positive in 10% of SLE cases with myelitis and approximately 20% of patients may fulfill clinical criteria for NMO.[30] The prevalence of aPL ranges from 18% to 60% in SLE patients with myelitis.[31]

Peripheral nervous system involvement may occur in 2–3% of SLE patients. Electroneuromyography (ENMG) can help identify neurophysiological patterns. Analysis of the CSF is useful in inflammatory demyelinating polyradiculo-neuropathy. Nerve biopsy can also provide useful information especially to delineate differential diagnosis. Mononeuritis multiplex is found in 33% of SLE patients with peripheral involvement, usually with subacute weakness in different nerve territories. It can occur at any time during disease course, either at the onset of SLE or later during its evolution.[32] Chronic inflammatory demyelinating polyneuropathy and acute inflammatory demyelinating polyneuropathy are relatively uncommon, being reported in <1% of NPSLE. Cranial neuropathies may involve the eighth nerve, the oculomotor nerves (third, fourth and sixth), and less commonly the fifth and the seventh nerves. Plexopathy and autonomic disorders are extremely infrequent.[19]

PATHOGENESIS

Diverse clinical manifestations imply that multiple heterogeneous pathogenic mechanisms singly or in combination contribute to disease process. Some of the postulated mechanisms for NPSLE include thrombosis, autoantibodies, cytokines and cell-mediated inflammation quite similar to pathogenesis in other organ systems in lupus.[33]

Autoantibodies are central to pathogenesis of lupus. Altogether more than 20 different antibodies have been detected in serum and CSF of NPSLE patients, which target brain specific and systemic antigens. Of these, focal neurologic manifestations are frequently attributed to antiphospholipid (aPL) mediated thrombosis via antibody-mediated thrombosis while, anti-ribosomal P protein antibody and anti-N-methyl-D aspartate receptor antibodies (NMDAR) are associated with diffuse NPSLE manifestations.[33] The risk of stroke or transient ischemic stroke in individuals <50 years is 8 times higher in aPL-antibody positive individuals than in those who are aPL-antibody negative. These antibodies are twice as likely in NPSLE than those without neuropsychiatric manifestations. Few nothermotic neurologic manifestations such as seizures, movement disorders, myelopathy and cognitive dysfunction are also linked to aPL antibodies. This suggests a pathogenic role for aPL antibodies beyond the thrombotic effects of aPL. It is postulated that thrombosis induced ischemic events in regions such as amygdala, hippocampus and frontal cortex may damage integrity of blood brain barrier and enable circulating autoantibodies and lymphocytes to enter the CNS. This may explain non-thrombotic associations of aPL.[34,35]

Ant-NMDAR antibodies cross react with anti ds-DNA antibodies and are associated with diffuse NPSLE especially when directed against NR2 receptor. High affinity cross reactivity between NMDAR antibodies and anti dsDNA has been shown to induce neuronal death by apoptosis in animal models. However, these antibodies can also be identified in non-NPSLE as well. Anti-ribosomal P protein antibodies are identified in up to 46% of patients with SLE. High tires are associated with psychosis, depression, seizures, coma, aseptic meningitis and transverse myelitis. Additionally, anti-aquaporin antibodies (AQP4), typically associated with neuromyelitis optica are detected in 3% of NPSLE patients. However, they were detected in 27% of NPSLE with demyelination.[30] Other autoantibodies implicated in pathogenesis of NPSLE include antiendothelial cell antibodies, antimicrotubule-associated antibody and antisupra-basin antibodies.[33]

The evidence for role of cell-mediated inflammation in pathogenesis of NPSLE is not robust mainly due to paucity of studies on brain pathology. Vasculopathy rather than cellular infiltration is the predominant pathologic finding in brain tissue. In NPSLE, intrathecal cytokine environment is swarmed by increased serum levels of multiple cytokines, including IFNα, IL-10, CXC-chemokine ligand 10 and CC-chemokine ligand 2 to name a few. IFNα seems to key role in pathogenesis of lupus and is demonstrated to be involved in aberrant synaptic pruning in a lupus-prone mouse models. Neuropsychiatric manifestations observed in this model were reversible with IFNα inhibition, indicating that IFNα is important in the pathogenesis of NPSLE. Synaptic loss in the brains of patients with SLE might be due to increased IFNα-induced microglial activation. Indeed, activated microglia are a feature of several mouse models of lupus and inhibition of microglial activation has been shown to attenuate the phenotype of NPSLE in murine models. Role of complement activation is an area of intense research in pathogenesis of NPSLE. In murine models of lupus, complement blockade has been shown to decrease the expression of inflammatory cytokines and adhesion molecule genes and diminish the caspase-mediated apoptosis.[33]

To sum up, the pathogenesis of neuropsychiatric disease in patients with SLE is multi-dimensional, complex and possibly unique to specific individuals or subsets of patients. The relationship between particular pathogenic factors and specific presentations of NPSLE remains unclear.

MANAGEMENT OF NEUROPSYCHIATRIC LUPUS

The management of neuropsychiatric manifestations of SLE requires a multidisciplinary approach. Investigations are chosen based on clinical manifestations. Apart from assessment of systemic lupus activity and exclusion of various differentials, attempts should be made to confirm diagnosis of NPSLE. Correction of any aggravating factors, symptomatic treatment and other non-pharmacological interventions are essential in addition to specific treatment for SLE. Symptomatic treatment is similar to other non lupus-related neuropsychiatric illnesses.[14] Mood disorders, seizures, headache and movement disorders are treated as indicated in non-lupus related illnesses. In mild cases symptomatic treatment may suffice. Non response to treatment or severe symptoms at onset warrants additional immunosuppressive treatment.[14,36]

Treatment is largely empiric due to lack of well controlled trials and is similar to other serious forms of SLE. Specific therapy depends on the manifestation with immune mediated/inflammatory processes treated with immunosuppression and ischemic processes treated with anticoagulation and antiplatelet agents. The distinction between the two is not always absolute and in a considerable proportion of patients both mechanisms may contribute.

MANAGEMENT OF INFLAMMATORY NPSLE

Steroids remain the backbone of treatment in most severe forms of lupus. The decision to treat with pulse methylprednisolone 1 g for 3 days depends on rapidity of onset and progression and severity of symptoms. Most of the reported series have used pulse methylprednisolone followed by oral steroids although lower doses may be equally efficacious.[37,38] The initial oral dose again depends on severity and usually ranges from 0.5–1 mg/kg body weight tapered over 3 to 6 months.

In most moderate to severe manifestations, cyclophosphamide should be considered although the evidence for its use in NPSLE is not as robust as lupus nephritis. A single controlled trial compared intravenous cyclophosphamide to intravenous methyl-prednisolone for the treatment of NPSLE. Methylprednisolone 1 g/day for 3 days was given as induction treatment in all patients. One group was treated with methylprednisolone 1 g/month for 4 months, then bimonthly for 6 months and subsequently every 3 months for 1 year. The cyclophosphamide group received IV cyclophosphamide as per the NIH regimen monthly for one year and then every 3 months for another year. Oral prednisone (1 mg/kg/day) was started on the fourth day of treatment and continued for no more than 3 months, and tapered according to disease activity/remission in both groups. Treatment response, defined as 20% improvement from basal conditions at 24 months, was observed in 94.7% (18/19) of patients using intravenous cyclophosphamide compared with 46.2% (6/13) of patients in the methylprednisolone group. No statistically significant differences in adverse effects were noted.[39] Observational data also lend support to the efficacy of cyclophosphamide in NP SLE. [40,41] It has also been used with success in paediatric lupus with neuropsychiatric manifestations.[42]

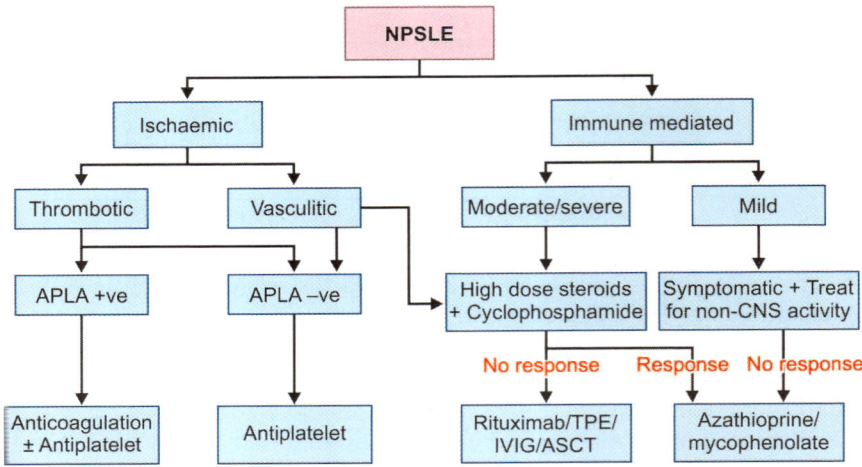

Fig. 9.2: Management of NPSLE

Mycophenolate mofetil is widely used as a first line agent for both induction and maintenance treatment in lupus nephritis. Trials in lupus nephritis have established its efficacy as non-inferior to cyclophosphamide.[43] However, very few studies have examine its efficacy in NPSLE. A retrospective observational series from India reported 88 patients with CNS lupus. Of these, 70 had inflammatory/immune mediated manifestations and were treated with MMF upfront along with deflazacort. Short term outcomes were favourable in 87% of patients.[44] An observational series of MMF in non-renal lupus reported good outcomes in 14/18 patients with CNS manifestations.[45] However, in view of limited data its use may be restricted to patients with less severe manifestations or contraindications to cyclophosphamide.

There is scarce data on azathioprine in the treatment of CNS lupus. It has been used for maintenance treatment after induction with cyclophosphamide.[40] In a series of 53 children with psychosis and cognitive dysfunction due to lupus 18 of 32 treated with azathioprine required a change to cyclophosphamide for poor response but none on cyclophosphamide required a change.[46]

Rituximab may be considered in patients not responding to standard immunosuppressive regimen. Tokunaga, et al. used rituximab in 10 patients with NPSLE refractory to conventional treatment. Most of these patients had failed cyclophosphamide. All patients responded to rituximab.[47] A series of 18 patients in pediatric NPSLE also reported favourable outcomes.[48] Intravenous immunoglobulins may be used in refractory NPSLE and in acute inflammatory demyelinating polyneuropathy (AIDP) where it is used as primary therapy similar to non-SLE-related disease. It is also useful when infection precludes the use of steroids and other immunosuppression.[49] Therapeutic plasma exchange has been used in refractory NPSLE. AIDP and myasthenic crises are other indications for TPE. Intrathecal methotrexate is another modality tried in NPSLE with good outcomes.[37] Autologous haematopoetic stem cell transplantation may be considered in patients refractory to all other therapies.[56]

MANAGEMENT OF ISCHAEMIC NPSLE

The management of ischaemic NPSLE depends on the presence or absence of antiphospholipid antibodies. In the absence of APL antibodies treatment with antiplatelet agents should suffice.[50] In the presence of APLA fulfilling criteria for APS, there is ongoing controversy on whether antiplatelet alone, anticoagulation alone or both should be recommended. Trials comparing low intensity to high intensity warfarin have not shown a difference in the rates of recurrent thrombosis.[51,52] Observational studies have shown the patients with APS with arterial thrombosis have a high risk of recurrence while on low intensity warfarin (INR 2–3).[53] Hence, a target INR of 3–4 or a combination of anticoagulation and antiplatelet agent is recommended.

In the presence of APL and non-criteria CNS manifestations associated with APLA such a chorea and demyelination, the optimal treatment is not known. In these situations the manifestations are considered to be direct effects of APL antibodies and usually respond to immunosuppression. Anticoagulation has been used with mixed results.[35] Primary thromboprophylaxis with hydroxychloroquine and aspirin is recommended similar to all APL positive patients in SLE.[50]

PROGNOSIS

NPSLE is associated with poor health related quality of life and increased morbidity.[54,55] A study from Netherlands found a significantly increased standardized mortality ratio of 9.5 (95% CI 6.7–13.5) as compared to general population. The most common cause of mortality was infection and NPSLE.[56] A study from Korea found a three fold increased risk of mortality in patients with NPSLE compared to those without NPSLE.[57]

CONCLUSION

NPSLE continues to pose considerable diagnostic and therapeutic challenges. Diagnostic workup and treatment decisions are typically performed on case-to-case basis. When considering individual patient care an important question to be answered is if the nature of the NP manifestations is thrombotic or inflammatory. It is important to include in addition to definitions, variables such as temporal relationship of NPSLE to SLE diagnosis, presence of disease activity, presence of autoantibodies, as well as favoring, and confounding factors. Immunosuppressant can benefit SLE patients with inflammatory NP manifestations, with significant improvement of quality of life, whereas, SLE patients with non-related SLE manifestations may benefit primary from symptomatic treatment.

REFERENCES

1. Pamfil C, Fanouriakis A, Damian L, et al. EULAR recommendations for neuropsychiatric systemic lupus erythematosus vs usual care: Results from two European centres. Rheumatol (Oxford). 2015; 54(7):1270–78.
2. Liang MH, Corzillius M, Bae SC, et al. The American College of Rheumatology nomenclature and case definitions for neuropsychiatric lupus syndromes. Arthritis Rheum. 1999;42(4):599–608.
3. Marc C Hoschberg. Updating the American College os Rheumatology Revised Criteria for the Classification of Systemic Lupus Erythematosus. Arthritis Rheum. 1997;40(9):1725–34.
4. Kassan SS, Lockshin MD. Central nervous system lupus erythematosus. The need for classification. Arthritis Rheum. 1979;22(12):1382–85.
5. How A, Dent PB, Liao S K, Denburg JA. Antineuronal antibodies in neuropsychiatric systemic lupus erythematosus. Arthritis Rheum.

6. Vivaldo JF, de Amorim JC, Julio PR, de Oliveira RJ, Appenzeller S. Definition of NPSLE: Does the ACR nomenclature Still Hold? Front Med. 2018 May 31;5:138. doi: 10.3389/fmed.2018.00138

7. Ho RC, Thiaghu C, Ong H, et al. A meta-analysis of serum and cerebrospinal fluid autoantibodies in neuropsychiatric systemic lupus erythematosus. Autoimmun Rev. 2016;15(2):124–38.

8. Mitsikostas DD, Sfikakis PP, Goadsby PJ. A. A meta-Analysis for headache in systemic lupus erythematosus: The evidence and the Myth. Brain. 2004;127((Pt 5)):1200–09.

9. Hanly JG, Urowitz MB, O'Keeffe AG, et al. Headache in systemic lupus erythematosus: Results from a prospective, international inception cohort study. Arthritis Rheum. 2013;65(11):2887–97.

10. Rayes H Al, Tani C, Kwan A, et al. What is the prevalence of cognitive impairment in lupus and which instruments are used to measure it? A systematic review and meta-analysis. Semin Arthritis Rheum. 2018;48(2):240–55.

11. Peretti CS, Peretti CR, Kozora E, Papathanassiou D, Chouinard VA, Chouinard G. Cognitive impairment in systemic lupus erythematosus women with elevated autoantibodies and normal single photon emission computerized tomography. Psychother Psychosom. 2012;81(5):276–85.

12. Kozora E, Arciniegas DB, Zhang L, West S. Neuropsychological patterns in systemic lupus erythematosus patients with depression. Arthritis Res Ther. 2007;9(3).

13. Alessi H, Dutra LA, Braga Neto P, et al. Neuropsychiatric lupus in clinical practice. Arq Neuropsiquiatr. 2016;74(12):1021–30.

14. Bertsias GK, Ioannidis JPA, Aringer M, et al. EULAR recommendations for the management of systemic lupus erythematosus with neuropsychiatric manifestations: Report of a task force of the EULAR standing committee for clinical affairs. Ann Rheum Dis. 2010;69(12):2074–82.

15. Appenzeller S, Cendes F, Costallat LTL. Epileptic seizures in systemic lupus erythematosus. Neurology. 2004;63(10):1808–12.

16. Kampylafka EI, Alexopoulos H, Fouka P, Moutsopoulos HM, Dalakas MC, Tzioufas AG. Epileptic syndrome in systemic lupus erythematosus and neuronal autoantibody associations. Lupus. 2016; 25(11):1260–65.

17. de Amorim JC, Frittoli RB, Pereira D, et al. Epidemiology, characterization, and diagnosis of neuropsychiatric events in systemic lupus erythematosus. Expert Rev Clin Immunol. 2019;15(4):407–16.

18. Abe G, Kikuchi H, Arinuma Y, Hirohata S. Brain MRI in patients with acute confusional state of diffuse psychiatric/neuropsychological syndromes in systemic lupus erythematosus. Mod Rheumatol. 2017;27(2):278–83.

19. Unterman A, Nolte JES, Boaz M, Abady M, Shoenfeld Y, Zandman-Goddard G. Neuropsychiatric syndromes in systemic lupus erythematosus: A meta-analysis. Semin Arthritis Rheum. 2011;41(1):1–11.

20. Hanly JG, Urowitz MB, Sanchez-Guerrero J, et al. Neuropsychiatric events at the time of diagnosis of systemic lupus erythematosus: An international inception cohort study. Arthritis Rheum. 2007;56(1):265–73.

21. Hanly JG, Su L, Urowitz MB, et al. Mood disorders in systemic lupus erythematosus: Results from an international inception cohort study. Arthritis Rheumatol. 2015;67(7):1837–47.

22. Palagin L, Mosca M, Tani C, Gemignani A, Mauri M, Bombardieri S. Depression and systemic lupus erythematosus: A systematic review. Lupus. 2013;22(5):409–16.

23. Jafri K, Patterson SL, Lanata C. Central nervous system manifestations of systemic lupus erythematosus. Ann Rheum Dis 2017;43(4):531–45.

24. Holmqvst M, Simard JF, Asplund K, Arkema E V. Stroke in systemic lupus erythematosus: A meta-analysis of population-based cohort studies. RMD Open. 2015;1(1).

25. Mikdashi J, Handwerger B, Langenberg P, Miller M, Kittner S. Baseline disease activity, hyperlipidemia, and hypertension are predictive factors for ischemic stroke and stroke severity in systemic lupus erythematosus. Stroke. 2007;38(2):281–85.

26. Sciascia S, Sanna G, Khamashta MA, et al. The estimated frequency of Antiphospholipid antibodies in young adults with cerebrovascular events: A systematic review. Ann Rheum Dis. 2015;74(11):2028–33.

27. Baizabal-Carvallo JF, Delgadillo-Márquez G, Estañol B, García-Ramos G. Clinical characteristics and outcomes of the meningitides in systemic lupus erythematosus. Eur Neurol. 2009;61(3):143–48.

28. Saison J, Costedoat-Chalumeau N, Maucort-Boulch D, et al. Systemic lupus erythematosus-associated acute transverse myelitis: Manifestations, treatments, outcomes, and prognostic factors in 20 patients. Lupus. 2015;24(1):74–81.

29. Fangtham M, Petri M. 2013 Update: Hopkins Lupus Cohort. Curr Rheumatol Rep. 2013;15(9).

30. Mader S, Jeganathan V, Arinuma Y, et al. Understanding the antibody repertoire in neuropsychiatric systemic lupus erythematosus and neuromyelitis optica spectrum disorder: Do they share common targets? Arthritis Rheumatol. 2018;70(2):277–86.

31. Alessi H, Dutra LA, Braga-Neto P, et al. Lúpus neuropsiquiátrico na prática clínica. Arq Neuropsiquiatr. 2016;74(12):1021–30.

32. Florica B, Aghdassi E, Su J, Gladman DD, Urowitz MB, Fortin PR. Peripheral neuropathy in patients with systemic lupus erythematosus. Semin Arthritis Rheum. 2011;41(2):203–11.

33. Schwartz N, Stock AD, Putterman C. Neuropsychiatric lupus: New mechanistic insights and future treatment directions. Nat Rev Rheumatol. 2019;15(3):137–52.

34. Kittner SJ, Gorelick PB. Antiphospholipid antibodies and stroke: An epidemiological perspective. Stroke. 1992;23(2):I-19-I–22.

35. Graf J. Central nervous system manifestations of antiphospholipid syndrome. Rheum Dis Clin North Am. 2017;43(4):547–60.

36. Magro-Checa C, Zirkzee EJ, Huizinga TW, Steup-Beekman GM. Management of neuropsychiatric systemic lupus erythematosus: Current approaches and future perspectives. Drugs. 2016;76(4):459–83.

37. Zhou H, Zhang F, Tian X, et al. Clinical features and outcome of neuropsychiatric lupus in Chinese: Analysis of 240 hospitalized patients. Lupus. 2008;17(2):93–99.

38. Franchin G, Diamond B. Pulse steroids: How much is enough? Autoimmun Rev. 2006;5(2):111–13.

39. Barile-Fabris L, Ariza-Andraca R, Olguín-Ortega L, et al. Controlled clinical trial of IV cyclophosphamide versus IV methylprednisolone in severe neurological manifestations in systemic lupus erythematosus. Ann Rheum Dis. 2005;64(4):620–25.

40. Fanouriakis A, Pamfil C, Sidiropoulos P, et al. Cyclophosphamide in combination with glucocorticoids for severe neuropsychiatric systemic lupus erythematosus: A retrospective, observational two-centre study. Lupus. 2016;25(6):627–36.

41. Neuwelt CM, Lacks S, Kaye BR, Ellman JB, Borenstein DG. Role of intravenous cyclophosphamide in the treatment of severe neuropsychiatric systemic lupus erythematosus. Am J Med. 1995;98(1):32–41.

42. Baca V, Lavalle C, García R, et al. Favorable response to intravenous methylprednisolone and cyclophosphamide in children with severe neuropsychiatric lupus. J Rheumatol. 1999;26(2):432–39.

43. Morris HK, Canetta PA, Appel GB. Impact of the ALMS and MAINTAIN trials on the management of lupus nephritis. Nephrol Dial Transplant. 2013;28(6):1371–76.

44. Gupta N, Ganpati A, Mandal S, et al. Mycophenolate mofetil and deflazacort combination in neuropsychiatric lupus: a decade of experience from a tertiary care teaching hospital in southern India. Clin Rheumatol. 2017;36(10):2273–79.

45. Tselios K, Gladman DD, Su J, Urowitz MB. Mycophenolate mofetil in nonrenal manifestations of systemic lupus erythematosus: An observational cohort Study. J Rheumatol. 2016;43(3):552–58.

46. Lim LSH, Lefebvre A, Benseler S, Silverman ED. Longterm outcomes and damage accrual in patients with childhood systemic lupus erythematosus with psychosis and severe cognitive dysfunction. J Rheumatol. 2013;40(4):513–19.

47. Tokunaga M, Saito K, Kawabata D, et al. Efficacy of rituximab (anti-CD20) for refractory systemic lupus erythematosus involving the central nervous system. Ann Rheum Dis. 2007;66(4):470–75.

48. Dale RC, Brilot F, Duffy L V., et al. Utility and safety of rituximab in pediatric autoimmune and inflammatory CNS disease. Neurology. 2014;83(2):142–50.

49. Camara I, Sciascia S, Simoes J, et al. Treatment with intravenous immunoglobulins in systemic lupus erythematosus: A series of 52 patients from a single centre. Clin Exp Rheumatol. 32(1):41–47.

50. Ruiz-Irastorza G, Cuadrado M, Ruiz-Arruza I, et al. Evidence-based recommendations for the prevention and long-term management of thrombosis in antiphospholipid antibody-positive patients: Report of a

Task Force at the 13th International Congress on Antiphospholipid Antibodies. *Lupus*. 2011;20(2):206–18.

51. Crowther MA, Ginsberg JS, Julian J, et al. A comparison of two intensities of warfarin for the prevention of recurrent thrombosis in patients with the antiphospholipid antibody syndrome. *N Engl J Med*. 2003;349(12):1133–38.

52. Finazzi G, Brancaccio V, Schinco P, et al. A randomized clinical trial of high-intensity warfarin vs. conventional antithrombotic therapy for the prevention of recurrent thrombosis in patients with the antiphospholipid syndrome (WAPS). *J Thromb Haemost*. 2005;3(5):848–53.

53. Ruiz-Irastorza G, Hunt BJ, Khamashta MA. A systematic review of secondary thromboprophylaxis in patients with antiphospholipid antibodies. *Arthritis Rheum*. 2007;57(8):1487–95.

54. Monahan RC, Beaart-van de Voorde LJJ, Steup-Beekman GM, et al. Neuropsychiatric symptoms in systemic lupus erythematosus: Impact on quality of life. *Lupus*. 2017;26(12):1252–59.

55. Jönsen A, Bengtsson AA, Nived O, Ryberg B, Sturfelt G. Outcome of neuropsychiatric systemic lupus erythematosus within a defined Swedish population: increased morbidity but low mortality. *Rheumatology (Oxford)*. 2002;41(11):1308–12.

56. Zirkzee E, Huizinga T, Bollen E, et al. Mortality in neuropsychiatric systemic lupus erythematosus (NPSLE). *Lupus*. 2014;23(1):31–38.

57. Ahn GY, Kim D, Won S, et al. Prevalence, risk factors, and impact on mortality of neuropsychiatric lupus: A prospective, single-center study. *Lupus*. 2018;27(8):1338–47.

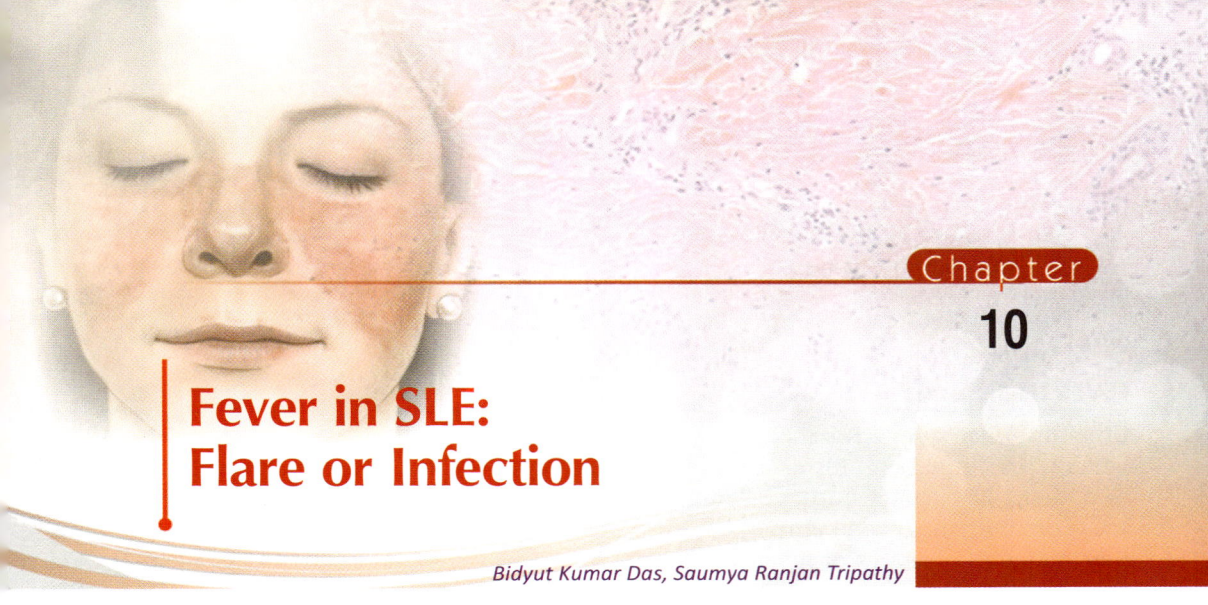

Bidyut Kumar Das, Saumya Ranjan Tripathy

Chapter

10

Fever in SLE: Flare or Infection

INTRODUCTION

Systemic lupus erythematosus is an autoimmune disorder which affects around 6.5–178 per 100,000 persons world-wide with an incidence rate of 0.3–23.7 per 100,000 person-years.[1] In India, the prevalence of SLE was found to be lower at 3.2 per 100,000 persons, though this data is nearly 25 years old and in recent times the prevalence seems to have increased.[2] However, increasing awareness of the disease and spread of rheumatology in India may increase the numbers if a current epidemiologic study is performed.

SLE is heterogeneous in its clinical manifestations. It can involve almost all organs/organ systems of the body. In a study by Cervera, et al. spanning 10 years with a cohort of 1000 SLE patients, the major SLE related problems included arthritis (48.1%), malar rash (31.1%), nephropathy (27.9%), NPSLE (19.4%), Raynaud's phenomenon (16.3%), serositis (16%), thrombocytopenia (13.4%) and thrombosis (9.2%).[3] One or more episodes of fever were present in 16.3% of patients. Complications over these 10 years included infections (36%), hypertension (16.9%), osteoporosis (12.1%), drug-related cytopenias (8.1%), malignancies (most commonly of uterus and breast) (2.3%). The 10-year mortality was around 6.8% with the most frequent causes being lupus flare (26.5%), infections (26.5%) and thrombotic episodes (25%). Whereas lupus flare and infection (28.9% each) were predominant causes in the first 5 years, thrombosis was the major cause in the latter 5 years (26.1%). Similar findings regarding infection were reported by Lifen Wu, et al. Infections were the second most common cause of death in SLE (25%) after cardiovascular causes.[4] Life-threatening infections occurred more commonly in the first 5 years of onset of SLE. In a recent review of causes of mortality in SLE, it has been noted that the major cause of mortality in developed nations is cardiovascular-related complications while infections remain the leading cause of mortality in SLE in developing countries.[5]

Case 1: A 28-year-old female, a known case of stable, mucocutaneous SLE for last 1 year, on 5 mg prednisolone and 300 mg of hydroxychloroquine daily, presented to the emergency with an episode of generalized tonic clonic seizures and altered sensorium, which was preceded by fever for last 10 days. Examination revealed altered mentation and diminished breath sound over the right infrascapular region with a pleural rub.

In summary, a patient of SLE presented with fever, pleurisy, seizures and acute confusional state. Investigation revealed leucocyte count of 10,000/mm³, platelets of 2 lakhs/mm³; ESR of 60 mm first hour, CRP of 45 g/L; C3 54.8 mg/dl, C4 14.5 mg/dl and dsDNA raised 1.5 times above normal limits. CSF examination was normal. The dilemma was, is it lupus flare or flare with infection. It is difficult to distinguish infection vis-a-vis lupus flare in such a setting with the currently available diagnostic tools, and therefore, there is a need for newer biomarkers that can differentiate flare from an infection. The current review aims to highlight the current position.

FEVER IN SLE

Constitutional symptoms including fever can be a presenting manifestation or part of the general presentation of lupus. Fever has been detected as a manifestation of SLE in 36–86% of patients in various studies.[6] Among patients with fever of unknown origin around 5% are ultimately diagnosed with SLE.[7] Although fever is a common manifestation of SLE, the percentage of episodes of fever attributable to active SLE is decreasing over time: around 86% in the early 1950s to only 41% in the 1980s.[8] The probable reasons for the decline in the percentage of attributable fever to SLE are use of steroids, non-steroidal anti-inflammatory drugs and increasing rate of fever attributable to infections, which are controlled by antibiotics.

Possible Causes

The differential diagnosis of fever in SLE is as myriad as manifestations of SLE itself (Fig. 10.1). Fever may be due to disease activity as mentioned above or due to infections which may be bacterial, viral or fungal in etiology. Further, infections can trigger lupus activity and thus both may co-exist as etiologic factors for fever in the same patient simultaneously. Apart from infections and lupus activity, other possible differentials for fever include coexisting vasculitis, overlap syndromes, macrophage activation syndrome, malignancies, or hypersensitivity to drugs.[6]

SLE Flare

The consensus definition of lupus flare as proposed by the Lupus Foundation of America is, "A flare is a measurable increase in disease activity in one or more organ systems involving

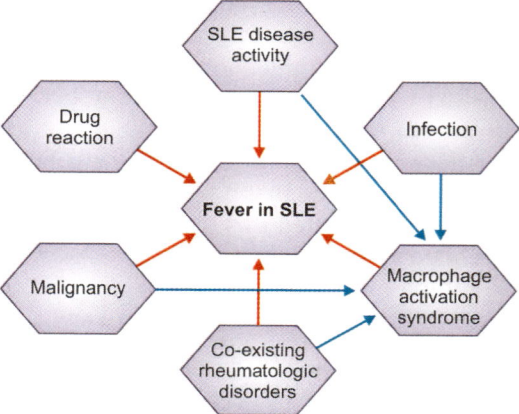

Fig. 10.1: Causes of fever in SLE

new or worse clinical signs and symptoms and/or laboratory measurements. It must be considered clinically significant by the assessor and usually, there would be at least consideration of a change or an increase in treatment".[9] However, the major problem in comparing trials dealing with the question of flare versus infection is the non-uniformity of definition for disease flare. Only a few trials have used the consensus definition for determining flare.[10, 11] In many trials, flare in SLE has been defined as an increase in SLEDAI score by 3 points compared to the previous SLEDAI score.[12–16] Others using SLEDAI to assess disease activity have defined flare differently the segment with SLEDAI >4;[17] SLEDAI ≥6;[18] SLEDAI ≥9;[19] SLEDAI ≥10;[20] SLEDAI ≥12 as a definition of severe flare.[21] Considering SLE to be a complex disease with varied manifestations, Rovin, et al. first divided SLE flare as renal flare versus non-renal flare and then divided each group as mild, moderate or severe flare with different definitions for each group based on BILAG definitions of disease activity.[8] Still, others have considered the opinion of the treating physician to define flare.[22–24]

Infection

SLE is a disease where there is an unfavorable immunologic state. On one hand, there is a predisposition to target own tissues and on the other, there is an impaired defense against infections. With this background, in the current era of biologics, where the modus operandi for treatment of SLE is by immunosuppressive agents: Steroids, cytotoxic drugs like cyclophosphamide, mycophenolate mofetil and ever-increasing exploration into the realm of biologics of which rituximab is the front-runner, there is increased propensity for infections. Infections mimic many clinical manifestations of lupus of which fever is the most important. Hospitalization rates in SLE due to infection range from 10–35% and results in mortality range from 29–53%.[10]

Burden of Infection in SLE

Bacterial infections account for 80% of infective episodes in SLE while viral infections account for around 14%.[21] Remaining infections include opportunistic infections including Mycobacterium tuberculosis. The most common sites of infection as per a recent study by Teh, et al. are pulmonary (37.9%) followed by septicemia (22.5%), urinary tract infection (11.8%) and skin infections (4.2%).[25] The most common organisms include Gram-negative bacilli (38.2%) of which *Salmonella* infections were the most common and Gram-positive bacteria (22.8%). Herpes zoster was the most common viral infection followed by chicken-pox. In other studies, urinary tract infection is the most common infection followed by respiratory tract infection.[23,26]

Macrophage Activation Syndrome

The differential diagnosis for fever in SLE is not limited to infection and disease flare. An intriguing situation which is now being increasingly recognized is macrophage activation syndrome. This condition can be triggered by infections, disease activity itself or malignancies in a genetically predisposed individual and is caused by an unregulated cytokine storm including the pyrogenic cytokines TNF-α and IL 6 and manifests as fever. The condition can be suspected in the presence of high-grade continuous fever, falling cell counts, increasing CRP levels and low ESR. High serum ferritin levels favor the diagnosis which can be confirmed by demonstrating activated macrophages engulfing precursor cells within the bone marrow. In a recent study by Gavand, et al. All patients with MAS in the setting of SLE had fever, and around 38% patients also had concurrent infection.[27]

Combination of Flare and Infection

The most challenging situation faced by every clinician treating patients with SLE is the simultaneous presence of infection and flare of SLE. Both conditions present with fever. It is easier to treat when the focus of infection such as pneumonia, urinary tract infection or culture-proven bacteremia is evident but in practical daily clinical practice, the site of infection may be occult. Besides, patients initially presenting with signs of infection may develop a flare of SLE triggered by the infection itself. Although the search for the unique test or marker which can distinguish infection from flare continues through decades, the all-or-none test is still elusive. Besides in most studies trying to distinguish between the two conditions, the number of patients with both infection and flare has been limited. There are few other studies which have clubbed such cases under infection for analysis. The current review is an attempt to highlight the differentiating points that can help distinguish both the entities independently when fever is a presentation in SLE.

It is vital to determine the etiology of fever on which the management of the patient and the outcome of the patient is dependent. In case of infections, it is essential to use appropriate antimicrobial agents and reduce immune-suppressants, while in case of a lupus flare increasing immunosuppressive dose is imperative to limit disease activity, limit organ damage and future morbidities.

DIFFERENTIATING FLARE FROM INFECTION

Clinical Picture

The first contact of a febrile lupus patient with the treating physician (preferably a rheumatologist) is very important. An intelligent, detailed history and clinical examination is imperative to detect the presence of infection, site of infection and also suspect the type of infection. It also helps in deciding further course of investigations. Although 60.92% of infections occur in the first year of lupus, there is usually no difference in age, gender, or duration of SLE in patients with and without infection.[28] Beca S, et al. had found that increased duration of symptoms and fever suggested flare while the degree of temperature rise had no statistical difference.[11] Patients with infection tend to have higher heart rate, and higher frequency of symptoms such as sputum production, vomiting, diarrhea, or abdominal pain whereas patients with flare had more frequent symptoms of arthritis, myalgia and cutaneous rash. They also observed that there was no statistically significant difference between infection and flare with respect to history of previous lupus nephritis or flares, including flares within last 3–6 months.

Use of Steroids

Most patients of SLE receive steroids at various doses depending on disease severity and many require a maintenance dose to limit disease activity. Rovin, et al. in their study on SLE patients under steroids developing fever demonstrated that at a median dose of 28 mg of prednisone (range 20–40 mg), fever due to SLE was completely suppressed within 24 hours.[8] In contrast, in the presence of infection, fever persisted despite the use of prednisone ranging from 35–300 mg. This suggests that in patients receiving steroids, fever should alarm the clinician about infection for which a thorough search should be made.

Investigations

There are some routine tests that support and certain tests that establish the presence of an infection. High total leukocyte counts with neutrophilia with the presence of left shift, high ESR and CRP are routine tests that suggest the presence of an infection in a normal healthy person. Cultures of blood, urine or other body fluids such as pleural, pericardial or ascitic fluid, CSF and pus directly establish infection. Some serologic tests such as IgM against viruses, bacteria like *Salmonella* or *Leptospira*, Widal for enteric fever, ICT for malaria also help in ascertaining the diagnosis. Imaging studies such as radiography, ultrasonography, CT scans and MRI scans help in localizing foci of infection.

Cell Counts

The hematological picture and response to infection in SLE are different from any other healthy person with an infection. The total leukocyte count and especially the lymphocyte counts are reduced due to disease activity and may not rise above normal upper limits despite the presence of infection. On one hand, the use of cytotoxic drugs like cyclophosphamide suppresses leukocyte production which predisposes to infection.[29] On the other hand, use of steroids often in high doses produces transient leukocytosis with neutrophilia.[30] Thus, in a case of active SLE under treatment with steroids and cytotoxic drugs, total leukocyte count and neutrophilia can neither be used to detect nor rule out infections.

Newer Tests Derived from Cell Counts

Neutrophil lymphocyte ratio and platelet lymphocyte ratio: In a study by Kim, et al. in 120 SLE patients with 60 patients having an infection and 60 patients having a flare, they found a neutrophil–lymphocyte ratio (NLR) and platelet–lymphocyte ratio (PLR) to be significantly high in patients with infection compared to flare.[18] Although certain other studies had shown higher NLR and PLR in SLE patients compared to healthy controls this study did not find any correlation with disease activity. A cut-off of 5.7 for NLR had a sensitivity of 75% and specificity of 90% in detecting infections and was better than high TLC counts and only neutrophilia. However, it was not as efficient as CRP alone and there was no significant added benefit of combining CRP and NLR. The study did not mention any cut-off values for PLR.

ESR and CRP

Erythrocyte sedimentation rate (ESR) and C-reactive protein (CRP) are non-specific markers of inflammation which increase in cases of infection, inflammatory disorders and malignancies. ESR increases in both SLE flare and infection besides being affected by multiple other factors such as age, sex and hemoglobin which makes it less useful in differentiating flare vs infection in case of fever.[31]

CRP, on the other hand, is not increased in SLE flares except in cases of arthritis and serositis. Multiple hypotheses have been suggested for the normal levels of CRP in SLE which include the presence of anti-CRP antibodies, suppression of CRP production and secretion by the liver by interferon-α and IL 10 which are increased in SLE, and polymorphisms in CRP (which may predispose to SLE).[31]

Ratio of ESR to CRP: To further elaborate the utility of ESR and CRP, Littlejohn, et al. studied the role of ESR:CRP. In their study of 53 SLE patients (28 flares and 25 infections), they found that for every unit increase of ESR–CRP ratio, there was a 17% increase in the odds of fever being attributed to SLE flare, after adjusting for total leukocyte count, SLE duration, sex, race and age. While ESR–CRP ratio and less than 2 was associated with 100% possibility of infections, an ESR–CRP ratio more than 15 was predominantly associated with SLE flare.[22]

Procalcitonin

Procalcitonin (PCT) is a precursor peptide of calcitonin and is produced by the C cells of the thyroid. Several studies have established its role in diagnosing bacterial and fungal infections but its role is limited in viral infections. Procalcitonin has also been shown to differentiate between bacterial infection and non-infectious causes of inflammation. With this background, procalcitonin has been evaluated in many autoimmune diseases including SLE, and most studies have demonstrated the role of PCT in predicting systemic bacterial infections. There has been a limited number of studies that analyze bacterial, fungal or viral infections separately. In the study by Shin, et al. serum PCT was higher in the group with bacterial or fungal infection (0.98 ± 0.12 µg/L) compared to lupus flare (0.24 ± 0.18 µg/L) or viral infection (0.13 ± 0.04 µg/L) and there was no difference between viral infections and healthy controls.[32] Similarly, Sahoo, et al. from India in their study on 75 patients with SLE, including 16 patients with flare and 21 patients with bacterial infections found elevated procalcitonin (≥ 0.5 µg/L) in patients with bacterial infection either alone or even in the presence of flare but normal in patients with flare alone.[33] A systemic review by Serio, et al[17] enlists six studies in support of the role of serum PCT in febrile SLE patients and suggest ≥ 0.5 µg/L as an appropriate cut-off for diagnosing infection. No correlation has been found between raised PCT and SLE disease activity as measured by SLAM or SLEDAI.

On the contrary, few studies have shown that PCT may be raised in SLE with concurrent infection and despite the presence of culture-proven bacterial infection, PCT may be normal at the standard cut-off of 0.5 ng/ml.[24] A meta-analysis by Liu, et al. included 8 studies with a total of 205 SLE patients in flare and 198 SLE patients with an infection found no difference in serum PCT between the two groups (pooled SMD = -0.45; 95% CI = -0.96 to 0.06).[34] However, subgroup analysis showed significantly high serum PCT in the infection group compared with SLE flare ($p < 0.001$) in the case of Asian SLE patients.

Traditional Markers of Disease Flare

Low complements (C3, C4) and increased anti-dsDNA levels have been used as a guide for the detection of flare. Many studies evaluating newer tests to evaluate infection versus flare have also evaluated C3, C4 and anti-dsDNA levels and tried to demonstrate differences between SLE with flare and active infection. Torres-Ruiz, et al. showed low C3, low C4 and increased dsDNA to differentiate SLE with and without severe flare.[21] Beca S, et al. and Kim HA, et al. showed a statistically significant difference between C3, C4, and anti-dsDNA levels between infection and flare.[11,18] Schafer, et al. found low C3 levels had 59% sensitivity and 77% specificity in detecting SLE flare whereas increased anti-dsDNA had sensitivity and specificity of 74% and 75%, respectively.[23] In the same study, low C3 was associated with disease activity only in the absence of infection while increased anti-dsDNA was associated with flare irrespective of presence or absence of infection. Yang, et al. had found low C4 and increased anti-dsDNA to be significantly different in flare versus infection while

C3 levels were similar.[13] On the other hand, Kim J, et al. and Chen CH, et al. had found C3 and C4 to be statistically different while anti-dsDNA levels were similar between flare and infection.[12,15] Similarly, Hussein, et al.[20] had found no statistical difference between dsDNA levels between flare and active infection groups and Pyo, et al.[14] had found C3 and C4 to be significantly lower in flare versus infection. Even so, the study by Wu, et al. found no statistical difference between C3, C4 or anti-dsDNA to distinguish between infections and flare.[4]

So, it is evident that there is a lot of variability in the findings and low C3, C4 and raised anti-dsDNA can only be used in combination to predict rather than diagnose flare versus infection.

NEWER INVESTIGATIONAL METHODS

Erythrocyte C4d to Complement Receptor 1 (CR1) Ratio

SLE is an immune complex-mediated disease where complements get activated. During complement activation, many complement degradation products are generated. C4d is one such product that binds mostly with erythrocytes and also with platelets and reticulocytes. CD35 (CR1) is a membrane receptor for C3b and C4b which removes activated immune complexes and gets degraded during the process. Both increased C4d and reduced CR1 have been shown as markers of disease activity in SLE. In a study by Chen, et al.[15] the ratio of erythrocyte bound C4d to CR1 was studied to differentiate the etiology of fever between infection and disease flare. Cut-off values of <1.2447 for C4d/CR1 ratio was 40.91% sensitive and 100.0% specific for the presence of infection while cut-off values of >1.2447 were 80% sensitive and 100% specific for the absence of infection in febrile SLE patients. However, the lack of standardization of procedures to detect C4d and CR1 reduce their clinical utility.

T-cell Subsets and Immunoglobulin G Levels

SLE patients with infection and flare were compared in a study by Wu, et al. and various lymphocyte subsets and immunoglobulin levels were assessed.[4] It was observed that in presence of infection, SLE patients had lower CD4+, CD4/CD8 ratio and immunoglobulin G levels while CD8+ cells were high compared with patients with flare. Although the findings suggest their utility in differentiating infection from flare larger studies replicating the same findings are necessary and these findings might just be predictors for infection susceptibility rather than the state of infection.

Risk Calculator for Differentiating Infection vs Flare in SLE

Beca, et al. studied 130 febrile SLE patients with fever attributable to infection in 48% cases and to flare in 45% cases.[11] 60% of these patients were randomly chosen to devise an algorithm and an online risk calculator based on days of fever, anti-dsDNA antibody titers and C-reactive protein levels to predict infection versus flare. The remaining 40% patients were used for validation of the risk calculator. The problem with such algorithms is that they are based on single-center studies and thus do not take into account racial variations and different infection patterns at different centers. Even at the same center, the risk calculator for flare in the inception cohort had an AUC of 0.92 (95% CI: 0.87–0.97) while the AUC reduced to 0.79 (95% CI: 0.68–0.91) in the validation cohort.

Delta Neutrophil Index

The fallacy of using total leukocyte count and neutrophilia as indicators of infection in SLE has been enumerated previously. Pyo, et al. hypothesized that the response of bone marrow to infections by producing increased numbers of immature granulocytes such as myelocytes, metamyelocytes and band forms may not be affected by SLE disease activity or drugs used for the treatment of SLE.[14] However, manual estimation of the percentage of immature granulocytes is tedious and observer-dependent. Pyo, et al. used an auto-analyzer with the feature of estimation of delta neutrophil index (DNI) which is a marker of immature granulocytes. DNI is estimated by subtracting the percentage of mature granulocytes from the percentage of myeloperoxidase positive cells. They found higher DNI to be an independent predictor of infection (Odds ratio = 18.9) and DNI >2.8% carried a relative risk of 8.48 for infection in a febrile SLE patient. However, DNI is a machine dependent result that may not be widely available and replication of similar results at other centers is required before it can be recommended for routine clinical use.

sTREM-1 and Pentraxin 3

Triggering receptor expressed on myelocytes (TREM) is a member of the immunoglobulin superfamily and is expressed on neutrophils and other macrophages in response to bacterial or fungal infection. Serum levels of the soluble form of TREM-1 (sTREM-1) have been shown to be elevated in infections. In the case of SLE, sTREM-1 was shown to be significantly high in case of fever with infection compared with patients with fever and SLE flare in a small study of 33 febrile episodes in 32 SLE patients.[12] At a cut-off of 53.2 pg/ml, serum sTREM-1 level has been shown to have a sensitivity of 1.0 and specificity of 0.664 to detect infection in febrile SLE patients. The difference in sTREM-1 levels between infection and flare persisted up to day 2 of hospitalization. In contrast, a recent study by Ajmani, et al. evaluating the role of sTREM in identifying infection versus flare in autoimmune diseases which included SLE and ANCA associated vasculitis and found no significant difference between infection and disease flare with regards to sTREM levels.[35] However, details regarding sample collection and duration of fever were lacking in their analysis. Larger studies with precise delineation of current symptoms especially fever and its duration, previous exposure to antibiotics and the day of sampling are prerequisites that may define the role of sTREM in differentiating flare versus infection.

On the other hand, a similar study by Kim, et al. failed to establish a role for pentraxin-3, a pattern recognition receptor to differentiate infection from flare in febrile SLE patients.[12]

2'5'-oligoadenylate Synthetase

2'5'-oligoadenylate synthetase (OAS) is involved in the type I interferon pathway which is an important pathway for pathogenesis of SLE. Considering OAS has many isoforms, there were preliminary studies by Ye, et al. which showed that mRNA expression of all isoforms (OAS1, OAS2, and OASL) was significantly increased in SLE flare vis-à-vis infection and normal healthy individuals; OAS1 was increased, OAS2 was equivalent and OASL was reduced in patients with infection compared with normal controls.[19] OASL correlated negatively with the presence of infection and performed better than CRP in predicting infection. Therefore, expression of OASL is a promising biomarker for distinguishing flare vs infection. But studies are limited.

Circulating CD27[high] Plasma Cells

Plasma cells are a major source of antibodies, and thus form a vital link in the pathogenesis of SLE. CD27, a member of the TNF receptor family when present on plasma cells enhances production of antibodies in response to various stimuli. It has been associated with the serological presence of autoantibodies in SLE including anti-dsDNA, anti-Ro, anti-La, anti-Sm and anti-histone antibodies. However, in a study by Yang, et al. which included four groups of patients: SLE without infection (n = 36), SLE with infection, non-SLE with infection (n = 8) and healthy controls (n = 26), they found that the percentage of CD27[high] plasma cells was high in both SLE with and without infection as well as in non-SLE patients with infection.[13] Comparison of SLE patients with and without infection showed significantly high CD27[high] plasma cells in the infection group versus those with flare (43.1 ± 6.3 vs 15.5 ± 1.8; p <0.05). Further studies with ROC analysis are required to establish a cut-off for distinguishing infection from flare in SLE.

Neutrophil CD64 Expression

CD64 or FcγR I is member of the immunoglobulin super-family and is expressed constitutively on macrophages, monocytes and eosinophils and few circulating neutrophils. On exposure to microbial wall components, complement degradation products and certain pro-inflammatory cytokines, there is a rapid increase (within 4 to 6 hours) in the expression of CD64 expression on the neutrophil cell surface. Hussein, et al. tried to evaluate the role of neutrophil CD64 expression to differentiate active autoimmune disease (24 patients with rheumatoid arthritis, 19 patients with SLE and 20 healthy controls) from infection.[20] The expression of CD64 on neutrophils was measured by flow-cytometry as the mean fluorescent index (MFI). The MFI (median range) of CD64 was increased significantly both in active autoimmune disease [36.15 (12–133)] and infections [49.0 (13–205)] compared with controls [5.35 (2.6–14)]. There was no difference between inactive disease and healthy controls. CD64 also correlated positively with disease activity (DAS score: r = 0.55; p <0.01 and SLEDAI: r = 0.51; p <0.01). However, it was also observed that increase in neutrophil CD64 expression was greater in the infection group compared with active autoimmune disease group and using a cut-off for MFI of ≥43.5 for detecting infection, the sensitivity and specificity were 94.4% and 88.9%, respectively.

The role of CD64 expression on neutrophils in distinguishing bacterial infections from active autoimmune disease (SLE- and ANCA-associated vasculitis) has been replicated by another study from India, where 51 patients with active disease (35 patients with SLE and 16 with ANCA associated vasculitis), 25 patients with bacterial infection and 20 healthy controls were enrolled,[35] The percentage of neutrophils with CD64 expression and MFI were measured. The mean percentage and MFI of CD64 expressing neutrophils (%, MFI) in the infection group (68.8%, 1037) was significantly high compared with those with autoimmune disease and without infection (7.7%, 456) and controls (7.0%, 99.5). Using a cut-off percentage as 30% for detecting infection, the sensitivity and specificity were 85% and 84% respectively.

Comparing the two studies, it can be inferred that neutrophil CD64 expression is a promising biomarker for determining and distinguishing infection from flare in febrile SLE patients. However, the method of detection and expression (percentage versus MFI) requires standardization. In view of the fact that mean MFI of controls in the latter study was higher than the cutoff MFI for detecting infection in the former study, using the percentage of neutrophils expressing CD64 may be a better alternative.

Table 10.1: List of investigations to distinguish infection from flare

Classic tests	Newer tests
CBC	Neutrophil-Lymphocyte ratio
ESR	ESR–CRP ratio
CRP	Erythrocyte C4d: Complement receptor 1 ratio
Culture (blood, urine and body fluids)	T-cell subsets and IgG levels
Procalcitonin	Delta neutrophil index (DNI)
C3, C4	sTREM-1
dsDNA	2'5'-oligoadenylate synthetase (OAS)
Miscellaneous (Widal, MP-ICT, Leptospira IgM, etc)	CD27[high] plasma cells
Imaging (radiograph, USG, CT, MRI)	Neutrophil CD64 expression

Table 10.2: Summary of relevant investigations to differentiate flare from infection in a febrile SLE patient

Test	Infection versus flare	Ref. no.
Neutrophil lymphocyte ratio	>5.7 for infection: Sensitivity—75% and specificity—90% in detecting infections.	18
ESR–CRP ratio	<2:100% associated with infection	22
	>15: predominantly associated with SLE flare	
	17% increase in odds of SLE flare per unit increase in ESR:CRP	
Procalcitonin	≥0.5 µg/L to detect bacterial infection	17, 32, 33
	No significant difference between infection and SLE flare except in Asian SLE patients	34
dsDNA	Increased dsDNA differentiates flare from infection	11, 13, 18
	Increased dsDNA: detects flare from infection with sensitivity—74% and specificity—75%	23
	Associates with disease activity irrespective of infection	
	dsDNA levels similar between infection and flare	4, 12, 15, 20
Complements	Low C3 and low C4 differentiate flare from infection	11, 12, 14,
	Low C3 levels: 59% sensitivity; 77% specificity in detecting SLE flare	15, 18
	Associated with disease activity only in absence of infection	23
	Low C4 only significantly distinguishes flare from infection; low C3 levels are similar in infection and flare	13
	No difference in C3 and C4 levels in flare and infection	4
C4d/CR1	<1.2447: Sensitivity—40.91%; Specificity—100% for infection	
	>1.2447: Sensitivity—80%; Specificity—100% for absence of infection T-cell subsets and IgG levels	15
	CD4+, CD4/CD8 ratio and IgG levels are lower CD8+ cells higher	
	No defined cut-off	4
DNI	>2.8%: relative risk of 8.48 for infection in a febrile SLE patient	14
sTREM-1	>53.2 pg/ml to detect infection, (sensitivity—100%; specificity—66.4%)	12
	No significant difference between infection and flare	35
2'5'-oligoadenylate synthetase (OAS)	OAS1, OAS2 and OASL increased in SLE	19
	OAS1 is increased, OAS2 is not affected and OASL reduced in infection	
CD27[high] plasma cells	Increase in infection significantly greater than increase in flare; no cut-off levels determined	23
	Neutrophil CD64 expression	
	MFI of ≥43.5 for detecting infection (sensitivity—94.4%; specificity—88.9%)	20
	% of neutrophils expressing CD64 ≥30% for detecting infection (sensitivity—85%; specificity—84%)	35

NLR—neutrophil–lymphocyte ratio; ESR—erythrocyte sedimentation rate; CRP—C-reactive protein; Complement 4d/ complement receptor 1 on erythrocytes; sTREM—soluble triggering receptor expressed on myelocytes; MFI—mean fluorescent index; DNI—delta neutrophil index

Table 10.1 enlists the classic and newer tests under research for distinguishing flare versus infections in febrile SLE patients. Table 10.2 summarizes the relevant investigations to differentiate flare from infection in a febrile SLE patient.

CONCLUSION

No individual test is yet perfect enough to distinguish flare versus infection in a febrile SLE patient. Clinical suspicion, traditional markers of flare (low C3, low C4, raised dsDNA) and traditional markers of infection (raised TLC with neutrophilia, ESR, CRP and procalcitonin) must be used in combination and the judicious decision by the treating physician. Although, the available tests and tools are not perfect due to several limitations and caveats, to distinguish infection and flare with a high degree of sensitivity and specificity, there is hope for the future. There are novel and promising biomarkers under evaluation that will help in bridging the current lacunae and provide a tenable solution to this practical problem faced by rheumatologists.

REFERENCES

1. Pons-Estel GJ, Ugarte-Gil MF, Alarcón GS. Epidemiology of systemic lupus erythematosus. Expert Rev ClinImmunol. 2017;13(8):799–814.
2. Malviya AN, Singh RR, Singh YN, Kapoor SK, Kumar A. Prevalence of systemic lupus erythematosus in India. Lupus. 1993;2(2):115–8.
3. Cervera R, Khamastha MA, Font J, Sebastiani GD, Gil A, Lavilla P, et al. Morbidity and mortality in systemic lupus erythematosus during a 10-year period: a comparison of early and late manifestations in a cohort of 1000 patients. Medicine (Baltimore). 2003;82(5):299–308.
4. Wu L, Wang G, Chen F, Lv X, Sun W, Guo Y, et al. T cell subsets and immunoglobulin G levels are associated with the infection status of systemic lupus erythematosus patients. Braz J Med Biol Res. 2018;51(2):e4547.
5. Ocampo-Piraquive V, Nieto-Aristizabal I, Canas CA, Tobon GJ. Mortality in systemic lupus erythematosus: Causes, predictors and interventions. Expert Rev ClinImmunol.2018; 14(12):1043–53.
6. TimlinH, Syed A, Haque U, Adler B, Law G, Machireddy K, et al. Fevers in adult lupus patients. Cureus. 2018;10(1):e2098.
7. LunchenkovN, Filippov E, Prihodko O, et al. Classic fever of unknown origin: Retrospective study in infectious clinical hospital. Open Forum Infect Dis. 2017;4:S343.
8. Rovin BH, Tang Y, Sun J, Nagaraja HN, Hackshaw KV, Gray L, Rice R, et al. Clinical significance of fever in the systemic lupus erythematosus patient receiving steroid therapy. Kidney Int. 2005;68(2):747–59.
9. Ruperto N, Hanrahan LM, Alarcon GS, Belmont HM, Brey RL, Brunetta P, et al. International consensus for a definition of disease flare in lupus. Lupus. 2011;20(5):453–62.
10. Mackay M, Oswald M, Sanchez-Guerrero J, et al. Molecular signatures in systemic lupus erythematosus: distinction between disease flare and infection. Lupus Sci Med. 2016;3(1):e000159.
11. Beça S, Rodríguez-Pintó I, Alba MA, Cervera R, Espinosa G. Development and validation of a risk calculator to differentiate flares from infections in systemic lupus erythematosus patients with fever. Autoimmun Rev. 2015;14(7):586–93.
12. Kim J, Koh JK, Lee EY, Park JA, Kim HA, Lee EB, et al. Serum levels of soluble triggering receptor expressed on myeloid cells-1 (sTREM-1) and pentraxin 3 (PTX3) as markers of infection in febrile patients with systemic lupus erythematosus. Clin Exp Rheumatol. 2009;27(5):773–78.
13. Yang DH, Chang DM, Lai JH, Lin FH, Chen CH. Significantly higher percentage of circulating CD27(high) plasma cells in systemic lupus erythematosus patients with infection than with disease flare-up.Yonsei Med J. 2010;51(6):924–31.

14. Pyo JY, Park JS, Park YB, Lee SK, Ha YJ, Lee SW. Delta neutrophil index as a marker for differential diagnosis between flare and infection in febrile systemic lupus erythematosus patients. Lupus. 2013;22(11):1102–09.
15. Chen CH, Tai SB, Chen HC, Yang DH, Peng MY, Lin YF. Analysis of erythrocyte C4d to complement receptor 1 ratio: Use in distinguishing between infection and flare-up in febrile patients with systemic lupus erythematosus. Biomed Res Int. 2015;2015:939783.
16. Bador KM, Intan S, Hussin S, Gafor AH. Serum procalcitonin has negative predictive value for bacterial infection in active systemic lupus erythematosus. Lupus. 2012;21(11):1172–77.
17. Serio , Arnaud L, Mathian A, Hausfater P, AmouraZ. Can procalcitonin be used to distinguish between disease flare and infection in patients with systemic lupus erythematosus: A systematic literature review. ClinRheumatol. 2014;33(9):1209–15.
18. Kim HA, Jung JY, Suh CH.Usefulness of neutrophil-to-lymphocyte ratio as a biomarker for diagnosing infections in patients with systemic lupus erythematosus. Clin Rheumatol. 2017;36(11):2479–85.
19. Ye S, Guo Q, Tang JP, Yang CD, Shen N, Chen SL.Could 2'5'-oligoadenylate synthetase isoforms be biomarkers to differentiate between disease flare and infection in lupus patients? A pilot study. ClinRheumatol. 2007;26(2):186–90.
20. Hussein OA, El-Toukhy MA, El-Rahman HS. Neutrophil CD64 expression in inflammatory autoimmune diseases: Its value in distinguishing infection from disease flare. Immunol Invest. 2010;39(7):699–712.
21. Torres-Ruiz J, Barrera-Vargas A, Ortiz-Hernández R, Alcocer-Varela J, Ponce-de-León A, Gómez-Martín D. Microbiological and immunological profile of patients with severe lupus flares related to bloodstream infections: a retrospective cohort study. Lupus. 2018;27(2):312–18.
22. Littlejohn E, Marder W, Lewis E, Francis S, Jackish J, McCune WJ, et al. The ratio of erythrocyte sedimentation rate to C-reactive protein is useful in distinguishing infection from flare in systemic lupus erythematosus patients presenting with fever. Lupus. 2018;27(7):1123–29.
23. Schäfer VS, Weiß K, Krause A, Schmidt WA. Does erythrocyte sedimentation rate reflect and discriminate flare from infection in systemic lupus erythematosus? Correlation with clinical and laboratory parameters of disease activity. Clin Rheumatol. 2018;37(7):1835–44.
24. Lanoix JP, Bourgeois AM, Schmidt J, Desblache J, Salle V, Smail A, et al. Serum procalcitonin does not differentiate between infection and disease flare in patients with systemic lupus erythematosus. Lupus 2011;20(2):125–30.
25. Teh C, Wan SA, Ling GR. Severe infections in systemic lupus erythematosus: Disease patternand predictors of infection-related mortality. Clin Rheumatol. 2018;37(8):2081–86.
26. Skare TL, Dagostini JS, Zanardi PI, Nisihara RM. Infections and systemic lupus erythematosus.Einstein (Sao Paulo). 2016;14(1):47–51.
27. Gavand PE, Serio I, Arnaud L, Costedoat-Chalumeau N, Carvelli J, Dossier A, et al. Clinical spectrum and therapeutic management of systemic lupus erythematosus-associated macrophage activation syndrome: A study of 103 episodes in 89 adult patients. Autoimmun Rev. 2017;16(7):743–49.
28. Hou C, Jin O, Zhang X. Clinical characteristics and risk factors of infections in patients with systemic lupus erythematosus. Clin Rheumatol. 2018 Oct;37(10):2699–2705.
29. Tian J, Luo Y, Wu H, Long H, Zhao M, Lu Q, et al. Risk of adverse events from different drugs for SLE: a systematic review and network meta-analysis. Lupus Science & Medicine.2018;5:e000253.
30. Shoenfeld Y, Gurewich Y, Gallant LA, Pinkhas J. Prednisone-induced leukocytosis. Influence of dosage, method and duration of administration on the degree of leukocytosis. Am J Med. 1981;71(5):773–78.
31. Dima A, Opris D, Jurcut C, Baicus C. Is there still a place for erythrocyte sedimentation rate and C-reactive protein in systemic lupus erythematosus? Lupus. 2016;25(11):1173–79.
32. Shin KC, Lee YJ, Kang SW, Baek HJ, Lee EB, Kim HA, et al. Serum procalcitonin measurement for detection of intercurrent infection in febrile patients with SLE. Ann Rheum Dis. 2001;60(10):988–89.
33. Sahoo S, Gomango BD, Goel KK, Parida M, Tripathy R, et al. Role of serum procalcitonin and C-reactive protein in differentiatingbacterial infection from disease activity in SLE. Int J Rheum Dis. 2017;20(Suppl. 1):101.
34. Liu LN, Wang P, Guan SY, Li XM, Li BZ, Leng RX, et al. Comparison of plasma/serum levels of procalcitonin between infection and febrile disease flare in patients with systemic lupus erythematosus: a meta-analysis. Rheumatol Int. 2017;37(12):1991–98.
35. Ajmani S, Singh H, Chaturvedi S, Mishra R, Rai MK, Jain A, et al. Utility of neutrophil CD64 and serum TREM-1 in distinguishing bacterial infection from disease flare in SLE and ANCA-associated vasculitis. Clin Rheumatol. 2019;38(4):997–1005.

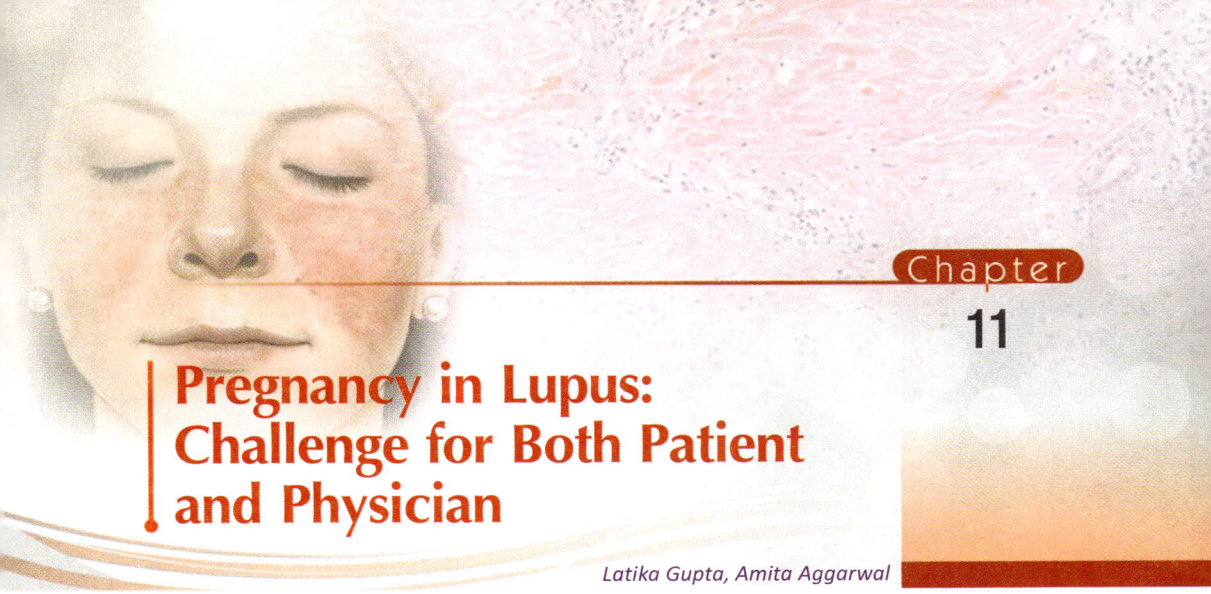

Pregnancy in Lupus: Challenge for Both Patient and Physician

Latika Gupta, Amita Aggarwal

Lupus is a multisystem disease, affecting young women, and consequently impacting obstetric outcomes. Therapeutics in rheumatology have come of age with better care and greater longevity, a pattern commensurate with better quality of life. Planning a family comes naturally to patients in such a setting. Changing societal structure, delayed age of conception, and smaller family sizes also mean that pregnancies are now more precious than ever before.

Apart from ethnic influences, access to healthcare can have a bearing on outcomes. Bridging the knowledge gap can improve treatment practices and patient counselling. A team effort is vital to deliver good healthcare in this challenging setting.

Case 1: A 24-year old lady was diagnosed with lupus 3 years ago when she had arthritis, malar rash and oral ulcers. She is asymptomatic on methotrexate 20 mg per week. She got married a year ago and now wishes to conceive. On routine tests her anti-dsDNA is negative and complement levels are normal. She is negative for anti-Ro as well as anti-phospholipid antibodies. She seeks, advice on the feasibility of conception at this visit.

This lady had minor organ lupus with a relatively uncomplicated course. Her disease has been quiescent for more than 6 months, a felicitous time for conception. The absence of major organ involvement precludes damage from the same, increases the chance of a successful outcome.

A diagnosis of lupus per se does not affect conception, unless cyclophosphamide or other gonadotoxic drugs have been received in the past. The only concern in her case would be the use of methotrexate, and the teratogenic risk it entails. She was advised to discontinue the same and avoid conception for 3 months from now to allow for complete a drug washout.

Planning a Pregnancy in a Patient with Lupus

Conception in lupus is best planned when the patient has been in remission for at least 6 months. A large observational study of 385 women found that 81% of women with low or moderate disease activity at conception had an uncomplicated obstetric course.[1] Another data set of 267 pregnancies stratified as per high versus low disease activity reiterated the same with a hazard ratio of 3 in those with active disease, although the number of live births was similar in the two groups.[2]

The patient ought to know that any pregnancy in lupus is high-risk, and entails risk of disease flare as well as poor fetal outcome. An initial screen for contraindications to conception is mandatory.[3] A mental flow-chart of the approach comes handy (Fig. 11.1). Preconception assessment includes evaluation of disease activity, antibodies that may affect the fetus, thyroid function, review of drugs and routine tests needed in pregnancy. All these tests should be done at baseline and repeated as suggested in Table 11.1.

After your advice she discussed with her family and decided to go ahead with conception. She returns to you with 10 weeks of gestation. She has consulted a gynaecologist near home and been tested for viral markers and TORCH antibodies. Ultrasound confirmed a single

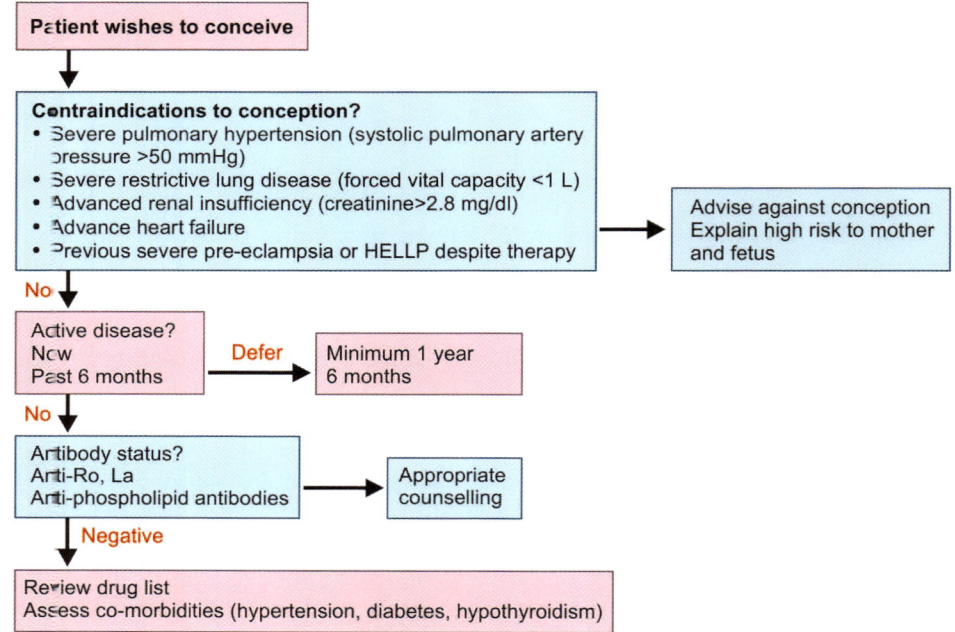

Fig. 11.1: Approach to a lupus lady contemplating conception

Table 11.1: Tests advised pre-conception in lupus		
At baseline	No nephritis	Nephritis in past
Hb, TLC and platelet count	Monthly	Monthly
Creatinine, uric acid	2 monthly	Monthly
Liver function tests, albumin, coagulation profile		
Anti-dsDNA, C3 and C4	3 monthly	2 monthly
Urinalysis		
If proteinuria is present, then protein creatinine ratio		
24-hour urine protein and creatinine	As in normal pregnancy	Monthly
ENA (anti-Ro and Anti-La), TSH		
Lupus anticoagulant, anti-cardiolipin, β2-glycoprotein I antibodies		

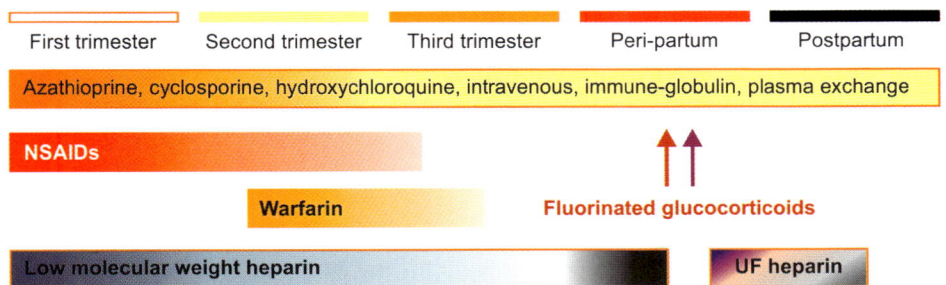

Fig. 11.2: Drug safety during gestation and peri-partum period

live foetus with normal growth. What tests would you advise her at this point and how frequently does she need to follow up with you?

Lupus patients should see the obstetrician monthly in the first trimester, fortnightly in the second and weekly in the third trimester. The physician should be consulted preconception and then once in 2 months if there is no flare.

They should get hemogram, liver and renal function tests done at every visit to the physician. If protein is present in urine, then 24-hour quantification may be done. Teratogenic drugs ought to be avoided (Fig. 11.2).[4] Patients with a past history of nephritis need to be watched more closely. Lupus nephritis affects obstetric outcomes adversely and, vice-versa, pregnancy affects renal function too.[5]

Disease Activity during Pregnancy

Hormonal changes in pregnancy exacerbate lupus and result in flares in 25–65% of patients.[6] Renal and hematologic flares are more common, although most are mild to moderate.[7] The risk of flares is further increased if patient has recent active disease or past history of lupus nephritis. Prolonged remission period before pregnancy decreases the likelihood of flare. Decreased flare rates in third trimester is reported in a recent study presumably because of blunted IL-6 response due to lower levels of estrogen.[8] One-third of patients experience flares in postpartum period.

Complications during Pregnancy

Pregnancy in the setting of lupus has higher obstetric complications such as pre-eclampsia and preterm labor, as well as disease related complications such as thrombosis, disease flare, and complications of concomitant therapy such as infections.[9] Fetal outcomes are also adversely affected as compared with pregnancies in healthy women. The concerns are heightened when there is recent active disease, or specific situation such as positivity for anti-Ro or anti-phospholipid antibodies.

Lupus with Anti-Ro Antibodies

Case 2: A 28-year-old lady was diagnosed with lupus 5 years ago when she had photosensitivity, oral ulcers and alopecia. Her symptoms are well-controlled on hydroxychloroquine 300 mg per day. She reports to you with a missed period and positive urine pregnancy test. On routine tests her anti-dsDNA antibody is negative, serum complement levels are normal though anti-Ro antibodies are positive. How would you advise her to proceed indeterminate?

Lupus has been inactive for a while in this patient, hence this a good time for conception. She does not seem to have organ damage to suggest any contraindications for the same either. She has not been on any teratogenic medications, another green flag for her. However, the only concern is the presence of anti-Ro antibodies, which entails a 2% risk of congenital complete heart block (CHB) or neonatal lupus syndrome (NLS).[10] Hence, we advise her to undergo intrauterine foetal cardiac monitoring beginning 16 weeks of gestation. The monitoring is done fortnightly to begin with and escalated to weekly between 24 and 28 weeks [11] In the face of prolonged PR interval on foetal electrocardiogram, injection betamethasone can be considered for accelerated pulmonary maturity. If there is hydrops or marked bradycardia then intrauterine pacing can be done for foetal growth. Hydroxychloroquine is the single most important drug that reduces risk of CHB, hence she was advised to continue it during pregnancy.[12]

Neonata Lupus Syndromes

NLS results from passive transfer of maternal autoantibodies (anti-Ro and anti-La antibodies) across placenta. Most infants a have rash which is photosensitive, and may get aggravated if phototherapy is given for neonatal jaundice. In addition mild anemia, thrombocytopenia and transaminitis may be seen. These abnormalities tend to resolve with the clearance of the antibodies by 3–4 months of life.[13]

Sometimes, the infants develop cardiac complications from damage to the fetal cardiac conduction system by maternal antibodies. The cardiac features include conduction defects, structural abnormalities, cardiomyopathy and congestive cardiac failure, the most common being congenital heart block (CHB). The presence of CHB often entails need for a pacemaker and at times even mortality (up to 15–30%). CHB affects about 2% of children born to primigravid women with anti-Ro antibodies though the risk increases exponentially to 25% in those with a previous baby with CHB.[10]

Lupus Flare during Pregnancy

Case 3: A 26-year-old lady had been diagnosed with lupus nephritis 3 years ago. She was successfully treated with mycophenolate mofetil then and has been on maintenance with azathioprine since remission 2.5 years ago. Currently she had been in remission when she received a nod from her rheumatologist for conception Her pregnancy was rather uneventful until the 24th week of generation when she noticed oedema in her feet, particularly worse in the mornings. She has noticed the need to get up at night to pass urine, and was also documented to have hypertension last week. Her bloods reveal a minor drop in haemoglob n (10 to 8.9 g/dl) and platelets (1.5 to 1.03 lakhs), while total leucocyte count was normal (4100, absolute lymphocyte Count 980). Anti-dsDNA antibody levels are 200 IU/dl while complements are normal. Urine dipstick is positive for protein (2+). Uric acid levels are 3.2 mg/dl. How would you manage the current situation?

The foremost concern in this patient is to differentiate pregnancy-induced hypertension (PIH) from a lupus flare (Table 11.2). The presence of proteinuria, high anti-dsDNA antibodies. normal uric acid levels are pointers towards a flare.The patient was started on amlodipine for hypertension and prednisolone was started at 0.5 mg/kg/day. In view of proteinuric relapse azathioprine was increased to 2.5 mg/kg/day.

Recognizing disease flare in pregnant SLE patients can be challenging. Physiological changes of pregnancy often confuse and confound. It requires more than just an astute physician to distinguish the two. Mild malar flush, arthralgia, fatigue and anemia is common

Table 11.2: Differentiating lupus flare from pre-eclampsia

	Pre-eclampsia	Lupus nephritis
Proteinuria	After 20 weeks	Anytime
Urine RBC or casts	No	Yes
Rash and arthritis	No	Yes
Seizures	More common	Sometimes
Uric acid	Elevated	Normal
Liver function tests		
Transaminases	Elevated	Usually normal
Albumin	Usually normal	Low
Complements	Normal	Low or declining trend
Anti-dsDNA	Normal	Elevated

in pregnancy and erythrocyte sedimentation rate can be raised. Up to 300 mg/day proteinuria can occur during normal pregnancy and liver synthesis of complements results in a rise leading them to remain in the normal range, even in the face of active disease. Thus, observing trends of various blood investigations carries more relevance than absolute values.[14]

The therapeutic armamentarium is limited due to the teratogenic risk in pregnancy, hence the approach is conservative and guided by severity of illness. Use of glucocorticoids is limited to lowest possible dosing, and flares tide over with short courses of higher doses.

NSAIDs can be used for mild symptoms with minimal increase in risk of congenital anomalies, and oligohydramnios in the late pregnancy. Hydroxychloroquine reduces flare rates and thus should becontinued throughout pregnancy. Azathioprine and calcineurin inhibitors have stood the test of time and are considered safe. IVIG and plasmapheresis remain alternative options in the acute setting but the higher risk of thrombosis with IVIG and fluid overload have to be considered (Fig. 11.2). Despite all measures, at times, one needs to use cyclophosphamide, which at times has been done safely in the second trimester.[15] Rarely medical termination of pregnancy to halt the autoimmune process is the final resort, when one is forced to choose the mother's life over the foetus.

She returned a month later with worsening hypertension, active urinary sediment and elevated creatinine. What would you do now?

Given the circumstances suggesting severe proliferative lupus nephritis and period of gestation beyond medical termination of pregnancy, she was counselled regarding the prognosis and the risk to foetus. She received methyl prednisolone boluses and injection cyclophosphamide monthly. In addition, injection betamethasone was administered for accelerated foetal lung maturity. However, she had a still birth after 3 weeks. Later her renal functions normalized and she achieved complete remission of nephritis.

Lupus with End-organ Damage

A 28-year-old lady with lupus presented with 6 weeks pregnancy. Her history was notable for long standing Raynaud's, pulmonary arterial hypertension and arthritis. Her recent echocardiogram revealed pulmonary artery systolic pressure of 55 mm of Hg. Her disease has otherwise been in remission after nephritis was treated 3 years ago, although she had persistently elevated creatinine (2.1–2.4 mg/dl) and proteinuria of 500–800 mg.

This lady has long standing lupus with concomitant renal damage. The ability to carry a conception successfully to term is significantly lower in the presence of chronic kidney disease. FAH further complicates the issue. This lady was advised medical termination of pregnancy which failed. She eventually underwent surgical termination with tubal ligation in the same sitting.

It is always worthwhile evaluating a patient for contraindications for pregnancy and advising appropriate contraception.

Contraception in Lupus

Despite the risks of unplanned pregnancy in the setting of lupus, contraceptive methods remain grossly underutilised. The inconsistent use of contraception in SLE patients may partly reflect limited screening, counselling, and gynaecology referral by rheumatology clinicians

The choice of the optimal birth control methods needs to be based on patient preference, risk from APL antibodies and possible medication interactions. Although barrier methods find widespread availability and ease of use, they are marred by a high failure rate.[16] Combined oestrogen-progestin combinations are useful in those with stable disease activity but caution is advised in those with APLs due to increased risk of thrombosis.[17]

Intrauterine contraceptive devices are safe and efficacious in lupus patients, although minor risk of pelvic infections exists. For patients who want to use a long-acting reversible contraceptive, the levonorgestrel containing intrauterine device (LNg-IUD) is an effective option for most patients with SLE and/or positive aPLs. Another advantage of the LNg-IUD is that it may reduce menstrual blood loss, which is particularly helpful for patients on anticoagulation. Importantly, progestin-only contraceptives have higher rates of discontinuation due to unscheduled bleeding.[18]

The vaginal ring is suggested to provide serum estrogen levels comparable to those seen with estrogen–progestin pills, but there are no data on its use in SLE patients. Women taking medications that increase serum potassium or alter renal function [such as angiotensin-converting enzyme (ACE) inhibitors], or women with renal insufficiency, require careful monitoring of serum potassium if taking drospirenone-containing oral contraceptives.[18]

Polypharmacy can interfere with drug efficacy, a risk most often seen with the combination of mycophenolate mofetil with OCPs.[19]

Lupus and Antiphospholipid Antibodies

Presence of antiphospholipid antibodies (aPLs) are present in about a quarter to a half of patients with SLE; although only a handful manifest with thrombotic or obstetric complications related to APS. All women with lupus and a bad obstetric history or arterial/venous thrombosis should be tested for the presence of aPLs (i.e. lupus anticoagulant, immunoglobulin G and IgM anticardiolipin antibodies; and IgG and IgM anti-beta-2glycoprotein I).

Asymptomatic carriers are women with positive aPL but no prior clinical event. Low-dose aspirin has been recommended but multiple studies have failed to show the benefit of this approach.[20] The second group includes women with recurrent pregnancy losses but no systemic thrombosis, termed obstetric APS. Combination therapy with aspirin and prophylactic doses of heparin significantly reduces the risk of pregnancy loss in this group. The third group is composed of patients with APS and prior systemic thrombosis. These women should receive full therapeutic doses of heparin throughout pregnancy. Heparin should be continued for 6 weeks postpartum. Low-molecular-weight heparin (LMWH) can

Table 11.3: Management of pregnancy with anti-phospholipid syndrome

Clinical setting	Antepartum	Postpartum
APS with prior arterial or venous thrombosis (irrespective of obstetric APS)	Therapeutic dose	Lifelong anticoagulation with Warfarin
Obstetric APS	LMWH and low-dose ASA	
Features of placental insufficiency or preterm delivery + aPL positivity but no clinical thrombosis	Prophylactic-dose LMWH and low-dose ASA Low-dose ASA*	Prophylactic-dose LMWH and low-dose ASA for 6 weeks Special attention to hydration and mobility, intermittent pneumatic compression and low-dose ASA while in the hospital. Graduated compression stockings and low-dose ASA for 6 weeks. For those undergoing Cesarean delivery, prophylactic-dose LMWH and low-dose ASA is preferred for 6 weeks
Laboratory aPL positivity but no clinical features&	Can consider Low-dose ASA*	

APS—anti-phospholipid syndrome, LMWH—low molecular weight heparin, ASA—amino-salicylic acid, APL—anti-phospholipid antibodies
*Can consider prophylactic-dose LMWH with low-dose ASA in refractory cases
& Based on limited evidence

be used in place of unfractionated heparin because it has comparable efficacy but fewer adverse effects with easier monitoring. Management of refractory obstetric APS is limited to anecdotal use of steroids, IVIG, and plasmapheresis[20] (Table 11.3).

Catastrophic antiphospholipid syndrome, vascular thrombosis and severe thrombocytopenia are reported in pregnant patients with antiphospholipid syndrome. Whether pregnancy increases these manifestations is still unclear.

Challenging Issues Faced by the Treating Physician in India

The culturally diverse and heterogenous population of India brings to the fore challenges unique to the treating physician.[21,22] While the urban set up is more reflective of what is seen in the developed world, patients from rural areas oftentimes bring in different issues.

Cultural beliefs dominate the mindset of lupus patients. Their obsession with influence of diet on the disease ensures that questions pertaining to that take precedence over all other important issues during the clinic visit.

Oftentimes, the physician faces a situation where the patient's kin bring her to the clinic, with glaring issues in medicine compliance and a request to keep the disease under wraps. At times the patient's in-laws come enquiring about the disease. For patients with juvenile lupus, marriage itself becomes a challenge. It is not rare to have a scenario where the husband is not aware of the disease.

Contraception usage is extremely poor.[23,24] Compliance with medicine intake becomes a problem. Financial constraints and lack of universal healthcare coverage is yet another constraint, which compounds the picture even further. Regional guidelines may be useful to cater to specific problems.[25]

To conclude, management of pregnancy in the setting of lupus requires the team effort of an informed rheumatologist, aware obstetrician and skilled neonatologist. Bridging the knowledge gap is vital to deliver good healthcare in this challenging setting.

REFERENCES

1. Buyon JP, Kim MY, Guerra MM, Laskin CA, Petri M, Lockshin MD, Sammaritano L, Branch DW, Porter TF, Sawitzke A, Merrill JT, Stephenson MD, Cohn E, Garabet L, Salmon JE. Predictors of pregnancy outcomes in patients with lupus: A cohort study. Ann Intern Med. 2015;163(3):153–63.
2. Clowse ME, Magder LS, Witter F, Petri M. The impact of increased lupus activity on obstetric outcomes. Arthritis Rheum. 2005;52(2):514–21.
3. Nahal SK, Selmi C, Gershwin ME. Safety issues and recommendations for successful pregnancy outcome in systemic lupus erythematosus. J Autoimmun. 2018
4. Knight CL, Nelson-Piercy C. Management of systemic lupus erythematosus during pregnancy: Challenges and solutions. Open Access Rheumatol. 2017;9:37–53.
5. Gianfreda D, Quaglini S, Frontini G, Raffiotta F, Messa P, Moroni G. Does pregnancy have any impact on long term damage accrual and on the outcome of lupus nephritis? J Autoimmun. 2017;84:46–54.
6. Stojan G, Baer AN. Flares of systemic lupus erythematosus during pregnancy and the puerperium: Prevention, diagnosis and management. Expert Rev Clin Immunol. 2012;8(5):439–53.
7. Saavedra MA, Cruz-Reyes C, Vera-Lastra O, Romero GT, Cruz-Cruz P, Arias-Flores R, Jara LJ. Impact of previous lupus nephritis on maternal and fetal outcomes during pregnancy. Clin Rheumatol. 2012;31(5):813–9.
8. Yasmeen S, Wilkins EE, Field NT, Sheikh RA, Gilbert WM. Pregnancy outcomes in women with systemic lupus erythematosus. J Matern Fetal Med. 2001;10(2):91–6.
9. Lee LA. Cutaneous lupus in infancy and childhood. Lupus. 2010;19(9):1112–17.
10. Brucato A, Frassi M, Franceschini F, et al. Risk of congenital complete heart block in newborns of mothers with anti-Ro/SSA antibodies detected by counterimmunoelectrophoresis: A prospective study of 100 women. Arthritis & Rheumatism. 2001;44:1832–35.
11. Buyon JP, Clancy RM, Friedman DM. Cardiac manifestations of neonatal lupus erythematosus: Guidelines to management, integrating clues from the bench and bedside. Nature Clinical Practice Rheumatology. 2009;5(3):139–148.
12. Izmirly PM, Kim MY, Llanos C, et al. Evaluation of the risk of anti-SSA/Ro-SSB/La antibody-associated cardiac manifestations of neonatal lupus in fetuses of mothers with systemic lupus erythematosus exposed to hydroxychloroquine. Annals of the Rheumatic Diseases. 2010;69(10):1827–30.
13. Penate Y, Lujan D, Rodriguez J, et al. Neonatal lupus erythematosus: 4 cases and clinical review. Actas Dermosifiliogr. 2005;96:690–96.
14. Lateef A, Petri M. Management of pregnancy in systemic lupus erythematosus. Nat Rev Rheumatol. 2012;8 12):710–8.
15. Férnandez M, Andrade R, Alarcón GS. Cyclophosphamide use and pregnancy in lupus. Lupus. 2006;15(1):59.
16. Andreoi L, Bertsias GK, Agmon-Levin N, Brown S, Cervera R, Costedoat-Chalumeau N, Doria A, Fischer-Betz R, Forger F, Moraes-Fontes MF, Khamashta M, King J, Lojacono A, Marchiori F, Meroni PL, Mosca M, Motta M, Ostensen M, Pamfil C, Raio L, Schneider M, Svenungsson E, Tektonidou M, Yavuz S, Boumpas D, Tincani A. EULAR recommendations for women's health and the management of family planning, assisted reproduction, pregnancy and menopause in patients with systemic lupus erythematosus and/or antiphospholipid syndrome. Ann Rheum Dis. 2017;76(3):476–85.
17. Gensous N, Doassans-Comby L, Lazaro E, Duffau P. [Systemic lupus erythematosus and contraception: A systematic literature review]. Rev Med Interne. 2017;38(6):358–67.
18. Toivonen J, Luukkainen T, Allonen H. Protective effect of intrauterine release of levonorgestrel on pelvic infection: Three years' comparative experience of levonorgestrel- and copper-releasing intrauterine devices. Obstet Gynecol. 1991;77(2):261–4.

19. https://www.mycophenolaterems.com
20. Corban MT, Duarte-Garcia A, McBane RD, Matteson EL, Lerman LO, Lerman A. Antiphospholipid syndrome: Role of vascular endothelial cells and implications for risk stratification and targeted therapeutics. J Am Coll Cardiol. 2017;69(18):2317–30.
21. Mohan MC, Ravindran V. Lupus pregnancies: An Indian perspective. Indian J Rheumatol 2016;11, Suppl S2:135–8.
22. Kothari R, Digole A, Kamat S, Nandanwar YS, Gokhale Y. Reproductive health in systemic lupus erythematosus, an experience from Government Hospital in Western India. J Assoc Physicians India. 2016;64(12):16–20.
23. Aalok Ranjan Chaurasia, "Contraceptive Use in India: A Data Mining Approach," International Journal of Population Research, vol. 2014, Article ID 821436, 11 pages, 2014.
24. Kumar M, Meena J, Sharma S, Poddar A, Dhalliwal V, Modi-Satish Chander Modi SC, Singh K. Contraceptive use among low-income urban married women in India. J Sex Med. 2011;8(2):376–82.
25. Kumar A. Indian guideline on the management of SLE. J Indian Rheumatol Assoc 2002;10:80–96.

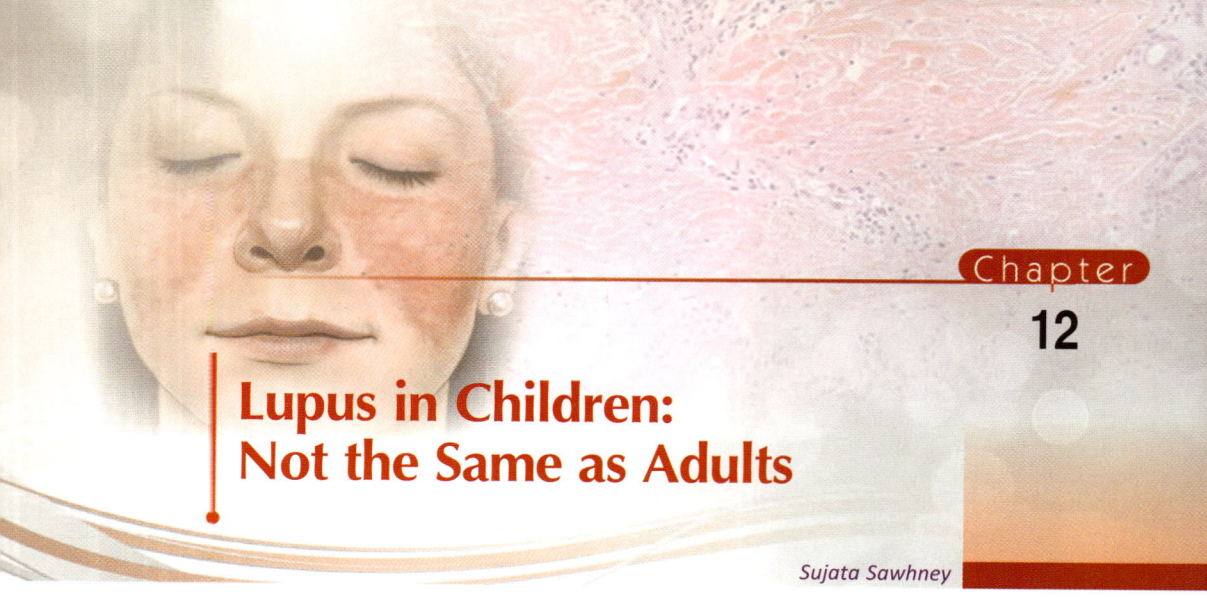

Lupus in Children: Not the Same as Adults

Sujata Sawhney

INTRODUCTION

Childhood systemic lupus erythematosus (cSLE) is the term used to describe lupus in patients with an age of onset less than 18 years of age and accounts for 10–20% of all lupus patients.[1,2] Lupus in children is not simply the adult counterpart starting at a younger age, but is in fact different in many domains: Epidemiology, recognition, presentation, disease burden, damage accrual and in disease outcomes. Lupus in children is a challenge to diagnose, manage, ensure adherence to the therapies, vaccinate and to transition to the adult services.[3] This paper will discuss the similarities and differences between adult and pediatric patients with lupus.

EPIDEMIOLOGY

There are differences in the incidence and prevalence of lupus across the world. The highest incidence and prevalence of lupus is in North America (23.2/100000 person-years and 241/100000 people, respectively) and the lowest incidence is in Africa (0.3/100000 person-years).[4] There is a striking race difference in this disease. For instance, in USA, the African Americans have a threefold incidence of disease as compared to Caucasians and also have a more serious and severe disease course.[5] Women are more frequently affected than men for every age and ethnic group. Incidence peaks in middle adulthood and occurs later for men. There is only one study on the epidemiology of lupus from India that estimated the point prevalence to be 3.2 per 100000 population.[6] Data from across the world suggests that the female to male preponderance is more marked in adults than in children.[7] A comparative analysis of 200 patients (100 adults and 100 children) from our center showed that the male to female ratio in the adults was 1:6 and in the pediatric population was 1:3. The median age at disease onset was 34 years in the adult patients and 9.4 years in the children, with a shorter delay to diagnosis in children compared to adults (0.75 versus 1 year).[8]

PRESENTATION AND CLINICAL FEATURES

The age of onset of childhood lupus is most commonly between 12 and 14 years, it is distinctly rare before the age of 5 and when it occurs early in life it should suggest the monogenic variety.[2,8] Children with lupus often present acutely with fever and cytopenias, the adult patient presents in an indolent fashion.[2,8] Children with lupus have an atypical presentation in 10–24% of patients, that is, they present with features not listed in the American College of Rheumatology (ACR) classification criteria. This can delay the diagnosis, the specific therapy and impact the long-term outcome as well.[5,9,10] Overall however, the delay to diagnosing children with lupus is less than that for adults, perhaps because the acute presentation and fever in the child provokes quicker medical consultations.[7]

In a study from our unit in India, 80% of children had fever and arthralgia at presentation and 25% had leukopenia.[11] Amongst the clinical features at disease presentation we found that children had more vasculitis, arthritis and lymphadenopathy (p <0.001).[8] The adult counterpart had significantly more thrombotic episodes and reported more fatigue.[8] Centres from across the world have reported more acute facial erythema, oral ulcers and photosensitivity in children as compared to adults. This could reflect ethnic differences in disease phenotype.[2]

Conversely, isolated discoid lupus in children is rare and tends to progress to systemic disease in 70% of patients.[12,13] This is different from the adult with lupus where isolated discoid lupus seldom converts to systemic disease.[5] Lupus nephritis is more common in children, 36% of children at our centre had nephritis at disease onset vs 26% of adults.[8] This is very similar to the report from Tarr, et al. from Hungary where 39% of children and 26% of adults had nephritis. The commonest class was reported to be class IV, with adults presenting with nephrotic syndrome more commonly than the children.[2] The adverse prognostic markers for renal disease such as proliferative nephritis, cellular crescents, hypertension, nephrotic range proteinuria, scarring and impaired renal function at presentation remain the same for both children and adults with lupus.[14]

We did not find any difference in the rates of neuropsychiatric lupus (NPSLE) in children and adults at our centre (24% vs 13% p <0.06).[8] There is a wide variation in literature of incidence of NPSLE likely due to different ways of assessing the disease and attribution to lupus rather than to infections, metabolic disorders or hypertension.[15] Children are noted to have cognitive impairment more commonly than adults. A meta-analysis of 16 studies that looked at the clinical features in adults and children with lupus was published by Livingstone, et al. in 2011.[16] The analysis included 16 papers that studied 5993 adults and 903 children with lupus and confirmed that of the clinical features of lupus, Raynaud's, sicca symptoms and pleurisy were the only ones twice as common in adults than in children. Another recent meta-analysis of more than 10000 lupus patients confirmed increased incidence of Raynaud's, pleurisy and photosensitivity in the adult patients.[17] In addition to overt clinical findings of various organ systems there is also a body of evidence accumulating that there are subclinical organ involvements such as ECHO abnormalities and pulmonary function test changes that should be screened for electively in children with lupus.[10]

IMMUNOLOGICAL PROFILE

There are no distinguishing laboratory features between adult and pediatric lupus patients. The diagnosis is suggested by a constellation of cytopenias, hypergammaglobulinemia, increased ESR and a positive ANA.[5] A comparative study from our center noted that the childhood lupus patients had higher numbers that were dsDNA positive and antiphospholipid antibody positive (p <0.001 and 0.02, respectively).[8] Similar findings have been reported from Canada where 39 cSLE patients and 165 adults with lupus were reviewed.[18]

CLASSIFCATION CRITERIA

There have been several classification systems used over the years: American College of Rheumatology (ACR) criteria 1982, modified in 1997, the Systemic Lupus International Collaborating Clinics (SLICC) 2012 criteria and most recently, the proposed new criteria from ACR /EULAR 2018, which are weighted in all domains.[19–21]

The SLICC criteria have been shown be more sensitive than the ACR 1997 criteria both at referral and in established disease for the pediatric patient with lupus. A study from UK evaluated the SLICC and ACR criteria in a cohort of 226 pediatric lupus patients and found the SLICC criteria to have a sensitivity of 92.9% versus 84.1% for the ACR criteria (p <0.001).[22] The specificity of the SLICC criteria is however lower than the ACR criteria: Children with hemolytic uremic syndrome and juvenile dermatomyositis can be incorrectly classified as pediatric lupus.[23] The SLICC criteria perform better than the ACR criteria for the adult lupus patient as well, especially in patients with early disease within five years from onset where the sensitivity of the SLICC criteria is 89.3% versus 76.0%; p <0.0001. This difference is lost in the late established disease of more than 20 years duration.[24]

DISEASE SEVERITY

There are multiple disease activity measures to assess disease activity in lupus: SLE disease activity index (SLEDAI), British Isles lupus assessment group (BILAG), lupus activity index (LAI) and SLE activity measure (SLAM). These measures have been shown to be effective for lupus assessment in children as well.[25] Children with lupus have a higher disease burden at presentation as reflected by a higher number of children with positive anti-dsDNA, low C3 and a high mean systemic lupus erythematosus lupus disease activity index (SLEDAI) of 16.59.[8] A Canadian cohort reported adjusted mean SLEDAI renal score was also higher in the children than in the adults (2.37 versus 0.82; p <0.0001).[26] Patients with cSLEare also reported to have a higher number of cumulative ACR criteria and a higher disease activity score SLEDAI (p <0.001 each).[7, 27] As the patients with lupus are followed up, the organ involvement accrues. In a study from a national registry in Portugal, where lupus patients were studied at mean follow-up of 11 years, skin, kidney, neurological and haematological disease were more common in children than in adults.The adults had more arthritis and increased percentage had anti Ro antibodies.[5,7,17]

LIPIDS AND BONE HEALTH

In children with lupus the lipid profile is proatherogenic at diagnosis and is impacted by both disease and prednisolone.[28] In adults, it is well established that the cardiovascular risk in lupus patients is six times that of the normal population and maximum in the 1st year after diagnosis.[29] Thus, preventative care to reduce the cardiovascular risk must be emphasized for the child and adolescent with lupus and patients should be assessed for hypertension, hyperlipidaemia, smoking, weight gain and counselled for regular physical activity.[30] Unlike adults there is no clear evidence that statins are useful in the pediatric patient with lupus. In the APPLE trial, the use of statins for 3 years to reduce the carotid medial intimal thickness in adolescents with lupus did not meet its primary end point. However, a subgroup analysis of the same patients suggests that adolescents with a high CRP may benefit. This requires further validation.[31] The prevention of osteopenia, osteoporosis and vertebral fractures is important for children on long term steroids.

Preventative strategies such as assessing the baseline bone mineral density, adequate weight bearing exercise, supplemental vitamin D and calcium intake and minimizing the dose of steroids are the backbone of care.[30] 35 to 50% of pediatric rheumatologists prescribe bisphosphonates to children on steroids, though calcitonin is seldom used.[32]

MANAGEMENT

The therapeutic principles and therapies available remain the same for all patients with lupus with an emphasis on avoidance of continuous steroids. If patients need long-term steroids to keep the disease activity under check it is far safer to use an appropriate disease modifying agent such as mycophenolate or azathioprine.[5] There is very little class I evidence for therapies for children with lupus and significant extrapolation of data from adult studies is used as a base for management protocols for children.[30]

As the disease burden is higher in children, immunosuppressants and steroids are used more frequently by patients with cSLE (p <0.001).[5,7,26,27] In addition to the 'medical care' that the children need, growth delay, adolescence and coping issues, psychosocial adjustment, adherence and finally transition to the adult services are unique facets that need to be addressed when managing children with lupus. These issues need to be carefully addressed with an empathetic approach via a multidisciplinary team.[5,30,33]

Some of these concerns are very commonly reported. Depression has been reported in up to 60% of children with lupus and self-reported medicine non adherence is 20%.[34] Growth failure needs careful monitoring and child's weight and height should be plotted on a growth chart every 3 months. The adolescent with lupus should also be counselled about contraception and fertility issues. It is generally safe for lupus patients to use oral contraceptives unless they are high titer antiphospholipid antibody positive. Finally, children with lupus should receive the human papilloma virus vaccine, pneumococcal vaccine and the annual flu injections.[30] Over a period of time co-morbidities such as diabetes, thyroid disease and hypertension occur with an increased frequency in adults with lupus.[7]

DAMAGE

Damage in patients with lupus is measured by the systemic lupus international collaborative index (SDI) and measures damage in 12 organ systems that is permanent and persists for 6 months. This index has been validated for children as well with some suggested modifications to capture child specific domains such as growth and pubertal delay.[35] Using the modified SDI 1,015 patients with juvenile-onset SLE in 39 countries were enrolled in a study. Of these, 405 patients (39.9%) had an SDI score of > or = 1 (mean +/− SD score 0.8 +/ −1.4). Renal damage (13%), neuropsychiatric damage (10.7%), and musculoskeletal damage (10.7%) were observed most frequently, followed by ocular damage (8.2%) and skin damage (7.6%). Growth failure and delayed puberty were recorded in 15.3% and 11.3% of patients, respectively.[35] The most important predictor for damage is ongoing disease activity.[36, 37] The SDI is typically higher in children with SLE than in adults.[26] In addition to more aggressive disease and increased use of steroids it could also be linked to an atypical presentation, that is, the presence of clinical features not listed in the classification criteria, reported in 26% from an Italian multicenter retrospective review. Such atypical presentations significantly delay the diagnosis and are seen in isolation in 10% of children. The most common is the febrile child with an acute abdomen. This study showed a SLICC damage score of >01 in 64% of children with atypical presentation vs 40% in the typical presentation p <0.004).[9]

The damage in the cSLE patient is inversely related to the age of onset of disease. A study from France revealed that younger the child the more the damage at long term follow up. This was attributed to several factors such as more severe disease expression, higher infectious susceptibility, and more aggressive therapy, particularly within the first 6 months of disease course. The SDI was studied in 56 children with lupus and was more than 1 in 89% of pre-pubertal cSLE, 57% in peripubertal cSLE and 38% in post-pubertal cSLE.[38] Data from Korea noted that there was no difference in SDI (p = 0.797) between adults and children with lupus.[27] Conversely, Tarr, et al. reported that the adult patients in their cohort had a higher SDI than children , however in this cohort the disease duration was much longer in adults (17 years vs. 6.9 years in children) and may have confounded the results.[2] A cross-sectional study from Portugal also reported that the damage was more in the adult cohort than the pediatric one, but this is not reflective of the cumulative disease damage that can accrue in the lifetime of the child with lupus and should be interpreted carefully.[7]

OUTCOMES

The overall survival of both adults and children with lupus is more than 90% at 5 years.[5] A meta-analysis of more than 25000 adult lupus patients revealed an all-cause standardized mortality rates (SMR) of 2.6 as compared to the normal population. The risk of mortality was significantly increased because of renal disease (SMR 4.689), cardiovascular disease (SMR 2.253), and infection (SMR 4.980). No increase in SMR was noted because of cancer.[39] A single center study from Korea that followed adults and children with lupus for 14 years reported a 2.9 SMR for adults with lupus but a 18.8 fold SMR for children with lupus.[27] The mortality in children with lupus is contributed largely by acute disease and infections, in adults the cause of death has been reported to be cardiovascular events and malignancies.[2] In a study of over 1000 patients followed for a mean of 7 years in Korea, the presence of hemolytic anemia (7.2, p = 0.034) and antiphospholipid antibody (aPL; 3.8, p = 0.041) increased the magnitude of risk of early mortality more in the patients with cSLE than in those with aSLE.[27]

CONCLUSIONS

Children with lupus are not just small adults. There are several differences in many domains (Table 12.1). Childhood lupus afflicts both boys and girls, presents acutely, often with fever and cytopenias and atypical presentations are also well recognized. Greater organ involvement and more frequent use of immunosuppression supports the concept that childhood lupus is a more aggressive disease than its adult counterpart.[7,18] Majority of the studies suggest increased organ damage in children with lupus. Attention to adherence, vaccination, growth and adolescent issues, reduction of future cardiovascular events, attention to bone health and finally transition to the adult rheumatology service must be addressed by the pediatric rheumatologist. Management protocols for both children and adults use the principle of objective assessment, limiting the use of steroids and aiming to treat to a target of remission in all disease activity domains. Following these principles of management, the pediatric rheumatology team can ensure that the child with lupus has the best possible outcome.

Table 12.1: Key differences between childhood and adult lupus

Feature	**cSLE	*aSLE
Female preponderance	3:1	6:1
Organ involvement	More acute, fever common, cytopenias and lymphadenopathy common. Increased renal disease and NPSLE	Indolent presentation, isolated discoid common, more thrombosis. Pulmonary, sicca symptoms and Raynauds common
Disease severity	Increased, more steroid and cyclophosphamide use	Moderate disease
Damage	Increased, related to aggressive disease and steroid use	Moderate
Mortality	Increased, more because of acute disease and infections	Moderate, more due to cardiovascular events and malignancies
Special needs	Growth monitoring, adolescence issues, adherence, transition to adult care	

*Adult lupus, **childhood lupus

REFERENCES

1. Barsalou J, Levy DM, Silverman ED. An update on childhood-onset systemic lupus erythematosus. Curr Opin Rheumatol. 2013;25(5):616–22.
2. Tarr T, Derfalvi B, Gyori N, Szanto A, Siminszky Z, Malik A, et al. Similarities and differences between pediatric and adult patients with systemic lupus erythematosus. Lupus. 2015;24(8):796–803.
3. Sawhney S. Childhood Lupus—Diagnosis and Management. Indian J Pediatr. 2016;83(2):146–55.
4. Rees F, Doherty M, Grainge MJ, Lanyon P, Zhang W. The worldwide incidence and prevalence of systemic lupus erythematosus: a systematic review of epidemiological studies. Rheumatology (Oxford). 2017;56(11):1945–61.
5. Papadimitraki ED, Isenberg DA. Childhood- and adult-onset lupus: An update of similarities and differences. Expert Rev Clin Immunol. 2009;5(4):391–403.
6. Malaviya AN, Singh RR, Singh YN, Kapoor SK, Kumar A. Prevalence of systemic lupus erythematosus in India. Lupus. 1993;2(2):115–8.
7. Sousa S, Goncalves MJ, Ines LS, Eugenio G, Jesus D, Fernandes S, et al. Clinical features and long-term outcomes of systemic lupus erythematosus: comparative data of childhood, adult and late-onset disease in a national register. Rheumatol Int. 2016;36(7):955–60.
8. Patel J AM, Shivpuri A, et al. AB0584 Paediatric vs adult onset systemic lupus erythematosus: The similarities and differences; a study from a tertiary care centre from Northern India. Annals of the Rheumatic Diseases. 2018;77:1445.
9. Taddio A, Rossetto E, Rose CD, Brescia AM, Bracaglia C, Cortis E, et al. Prognostic impact of atypical presentation in pediatric systemic lupus erythematosus: Results from a multicenter study. J Pediatr. 2010;156(6):972–7.
10. Huggins JL, Holland MJ, Brunner HI. Organ involvement other than lupus nephritis in childhood-onset systemic lupus erythematosus. Lupus. 2016;25(8):857–63.
11. Sawhney S, Jariwala M, Agarwal M. A77: Clinical and laboratory features and systemic lupus erythematous disease activity index 2000 (SLEDAI 2K) at onset and follow-up in a cohort of 109 paediatric lupus patients from a tertiary level centre in India. Arthritis and Rheumatology. 2014; 66(S3):S109–S10.
12. George PM, Tunnessen WW, Jr. Childhood discoid lupus erythematosus. Arch Dermatol. 1993; 129(5):613–7.
13. Arkin LM, Ansell L, Rademaker A, Curran ML, Miller ML, Wagner A, et al. The natural history of pediatric-onset discoid lupus erythematosus. J Am Acad Dermatol. 2015;72(4):628–33.

14. Baqi N, Moazami S, Singh A, Ahmad H, Balachandra S, Tejani A. Lupus nephritis in children: A longitudinal study of prognostic factors and therapy. J Am Soc Nephrol. 1996;7(6):924–9.
15. Postal M, Costallat LT, Appenzeller S. Neuropsychiatric manifestations in systemic lupus erythematosus: Epidemiology, pathophysiology and management. CNS Drugs. 2011;25(9):721–36.
16. Livingston B, Bonner A, Pope J. Differences in clinical manifestations between childhood-onset lupus and adult-onset lupus: A meta-analysis. Lupus. 2011;20(13):1345–55.
17. Bundhun PK, Kumari A, Huang F. Differences in clinical features observed between childhood-onset versus adult-onset systemic lupus erythematosus: A systematic review and meta-analysis. Medicine (Baltimore). 2017;96(37):e8086.
18. Tucker LB, Menon S, Schaller JG, Isenberg DA. Adult- and childhood-onset systemic lupus erythematosus: a comparison of onset, clinical features, serology, and outcome. Br J Rheumatol. 1995;34(9):866–72.
19. Petri M, Orbai AM, Alarcon GS, Gordon C, Merrill JT, Fortin PR, et al. Derivation and validation of the Systemic Lupus International Collaborating Clinics classification criteria for systemic lupus erythematosus. Arthritis Rheum. 2012;64(8):2677–86.
20. Aringer M, Dorner T, Leuchten N, Johnson SR. Toward new criteria for systemic lupus erythematosus- a standpoint. Lupus. 2016;25(8):805–11.
21. Hochberg MC. Updating the American College of Rheumatology revised criteria for the classification of systemic lupus erythematosus. Arthritis Rheum. 1997;40(9):1725.
22. Lythgoe H, Morgan T, Heaf E, Lloyd O, Al-Abadi E, Armon K, et al. Evaluation of the ACR and SLICC classification criteria in juvenile-onset systemic lupus erythematosus: A longitudinal analysis. Lupus. 2017;26(12):1285–90.
23. Sag E, Tartaglione A, Batu ED, Ravelli A, Khalil SM, Marks SD, et al. Performance of the new SLICC classification criteria in childhood systemic lupus erythematosus: A multicentre study. Clin Exp Rheumatol. 2014;32(3):440–4.
24. Ines L, Silva C, Galindo M, Lopez-Longo FJ, Terroso G, Romao VC, et al. Classification of Systemic Lupus Erythematosus: Systemic Lupus International Collaborating Clinics Versus American College of Rheumatology Criteria. A Comparative Study of 2,055 Patients From a Real-Life, International Systemic Lupus Erythematosus Cohort. Arthritis Care Res (Hoboken). 2015;67(8):1180–5.
25. Brunner HI, Feldman BM, Bombardier C, Silverman ED. Sensitivity of the Systemic Lupus Erythematosus Disease Activity Index, British Isles Lupus Assessment Group Index, and Systemic Lupus Activity Measure in the evaluation of clinical change in childhood-onset systemic lupus erythematosus. Arthritis Rheum. 1999;42(7):1354–60.
26. Brunner HI, Gladman DD, Ibanez D, Urowitz MD, Silverman ED. Difference in disease features between childhood-onset and adult-onset systemic lupus erythematosus. Arthritis Rheum. 2008;58(2):556–62.
27. Joo YB, Park SY, Won S, Bae SC. Differences in clinical features and mortality between childhood-onset and adult-onset systemic lupus erythematosus: A prospective single-center study. J Rheumatol. 2016;43(8):1490–7.
28. Sarkissian T, Beyene J, Feldman B, McCrindle B, Silverman ED. Longitudinal examination of lipid profiles in pediatric systemic lupus erythematosus. Arthritis Rheum. 2007;56(2):631–8.
29. Avina-Zubieta JA, To F, Vostretsova K, De Vera M, Sayre EC, Esdaile JM. Risk of myocardial infarction and stroke in newly diagnosed systemic lupus erythematosus: A general population-based study. Arthritis Care Res (Hoboken). 2017;69(6):849–56.
30. Morgan TA, Watson L, McCann LJ, Beresford MW. Children and adolescents with SLE: Not just little adults. Lupus. 2013;22(12):1309–19.
31. Ardoin SP, Schanberg LE, Sandborg CI, Barnhart HX, Evans GW, Yow E, et al. Secondary analysis of APPLE study suggests atorvastatin may reduce atherosclerosis progression in pubertal lupus patients with higher C reactive protein. Ann Rheum Dis. 2014;73(3):557–66.
32. Soybilgic A, Tesher M, Wagner-Weiner L, Onel KB. A survey of steroid-related osteoporosis diagnosis, prevention and treatment practices of pediatric rheumatologists in North America. Pediatr Rheumatol Online J. 2014;12:24.
33. Aggarwal A, Srivastava P. Childhood onset systemic lupus erythematosus: How is it different from adult SLE? Int J Rheum Dis. 2015;18(2):182–91.

34. Davis AM, Graham TB, Zhu Y, McPheeters ML. Depression and medication nonadherence in childhood-onset systemic lupus erythematosus. Lupus. 2018;27(9):1532–41.

35. Gutierrez-Suarez R, Ruperto N, Gastaldi R, Pistorio A, Felici E, Burgos-Vargas R, et al. A proposal for a pediatric version of the systemic lupus international collaborating clinics/American College of Rheumatology Damage Index based on the analysis of 1,015 patients with juvenile-onset systemic lupus erythematosus. Arthritis Rheum. 2006;54(9):2989–96.

36. Stoll T, Sutcliffe N, Mach J, Klaghofer R, Isenberg DA. Analysis of the relationship between disease activity and damage in patients with systemic lupus erythematosus—a 5-yr prospective study. Rheumatology (Oxford). 2004;43(8):1039–44.

37. Hiraki LT, Hamilton J, Silverman ED. Measuring permanent damage in pediatric systemic lupus erythematosus. Lupus. 2007;16(8):657–62.

38. Descloux E, Durieu I, Cochat P, Vital-Durand D, Ninet J, Fabien N, et al. Influence of age at disease onset in the outcome of paediatric systemic lupus erythematosus. Rheumatology (Oxford). 2009;48(7):779–84.

39. Lee YH, Choi SJ, Ji JD, Song GG. Overall and cause-specific mortality in systemic lupus erythematosus: An updated meta-analysis. Lupus. 2016;25(7):727–34.

Management of Lupus: Balancing Risks and Benefits

Keerthi Talari Bommakanti, Liza Rajasekhar

INTRODUCTION

Managing lupus in 2020 is all about balancing the risks of treatment with its benefits. Over the last five decades, survival rates in lupus have improved from a 5-year survival of 50% in 1950 to a 10-year survival of 85% reflecting the benefits of treatment of lupus. From the individual patient's perspective there are still many questions about how safe these treatment options are in the short-term and long-term. Physicians are aware that therapies in lupus entail some reversible and some irreversible side-effects. In the absence of any major breakthrough in the management of lupus it falls upon the medical fraternity to choose the path which balances the risks and benefits of treatment.

There is a lacuna in the progress of new treatment options for lupus. While treat to target is now the standard approach in rheumatoid arthritis, it is not so in SLE. This is primarily related to multiorgan involvement, varying severity, damage accrual, drug toxicity, associated fatigue and depression. With failure of most of the biologics in lupus, it seems that we need to use current drugs judiciously. This review outlines the benefits of current practises in lupus management and the risks that are associated with the same and a proposal on how to balance the risk and the benefit.

Case 1: A 29-year-old newly married male patient was diagnosed to have SLE after 2 years of symptoms which included inflammatory polyarthritis, psoriasiform scaly rash over the scalp and later development of fever of unknown origin. After initiating on hydroxychloroquine and mycophenolate mofetil he complained of severe upper abdominal pain, relating it to hydroxychloroquine. Extensive evaluation of ongoing fever did not reveal any infection and immunosuppression was continued. Cytopenia's and transaminitis developed and he was treated with high dose steroids considering macrophage activation syndrome of lupus. He refused cyclophosphamide and rituximab. Fever and laboratory abnormalities subsided. He reported anxiety, insomnia and abdominal cramps. He was initiated on treatment of anxiety disorder and improved. Over the next 2 years he had mild flares in the form of arthritis and malar rash and complied with 2.5 g daily of mycophenolate, low dose steroid and hydroxychloquine. He was overjoyed to become a father. Evaluation of a recent onset unilateral hip pain revealed avascular necrosis at both hips. This case highlights that the drugs that we use not only give substantial benefit but also have potential risks.

BENEFITS

Management of lupus involves induction of remission and then maintaining the disease remission. Monitoring at regular intervals helps in detection of flares at an early stage. Data suggests that fewer the number of flares and earlier the control of disease activity, less is the long-term damage. Also, regular follow-up gives us an opportunity to understand the patient's mental and emotional status at that time point which helps in counselling them accordingly. This prevents non-compliance, fatigue and depression which otherwise would adversely affect the quality of life of the patient.

However, the heterogeneity in lupus management is obvious as a literature search revealed 2399 articles on guidelines and consensus statements in lupus management. In this systematic review, out of these 2399 articles, 14 articles, 9 guidelines and 6 consensus statements were included. Most of the guidelines focussed on the management of lupus nephritis, few of them on neuropsychiatric lupus while only 2 of them spoke about the management of other manifestations which was also not supported by adequate evidence.[1]

Constitutional manifestations are usually managed with antimalarial drugs, corticosteroids, and non-steroidal anti-inflammatory drugs. Arthritis which on occasion can overshadow other manifestations of lupus is managed with corticosteroids, antimalarial drugs, methotrexate and azathioprine, and for refractory disease, mycophenolate mofetil as well as rituximab may also be considered. Corticosteroids, azathioprine, mycophenolate, or cyclophosphamide are recommended for hematologic manifestations, with rituximab and plasma exchange recommended in refractory disease. Splenectomy may be considered when all else fails. These recommendations are based either on expert opinion or prospective, observational data but not on randomised controlled trials. Treatment for neuropsychiatric lupus was discussed in two EULAR guidelines.[2,3] For manifestations like acute confusional state, movement disorders, myelitis, psychosis, optic neuritis or peripheral neuropathy induction therapy (high-dose corticosteroids and intravenous cyclophosphamide) followed with maintenance therapy is recommended while cerebrovascular accident, cognitive dysfunction, seizures, and major depression are recommended to be managed as for the general population. Anticoagulation is to be added for patients with associated antiphospholipid antibody syndrome. Rituximab for cognitive deficits, psychosis, or seizures and IV immunoglobulin or plasmapheresis for refractory disease has been suggested. Except for intravenous cyclophosphamide in neuropsychiatric lupus, no medication is backed by a controlled trial. Even in the trial of cyclophosphamide versus steroids for neuropsychiatric lupus, only 32 patients were randomised and a 20% improvement of clinical symptoms was considered as response.[4]

Maximum evidence is available for lupus nephritis and the recommendations as per different guidelines are summarised in Table 13.1.[5–7] Most of the guidelines concur except for recommendations for when to biopsy, treatment of class II LN, first line for class V LN and on assessing the response to treatment. In most of the trials on cyclophosphamide or mycophenolate for induction complete response was observed in around 40% of patients with lupus nephritis with partial response in another 20%.

Hydroxychloroquine is recommended for all patients with lupus. While originally, it was used for cutaneous and articular manifestations of lupus, it has been later on found to decrease flare rates, decrease damage accrual and improve survival. It has also been found to improve insulin resistance, decrease cholesterol and has antithrombotic effects. Hydroxychloroquine also improves pregnancy outcomes with fewer flares, more successful

Table 13.1: Recommendations in management of lupus nephritis

Recommendation	EULAR-ERA EDTA[5]	ACR[6]	KDIGO[7]
Indication for renal biopsy	>0.5 g/day proteinuria with or without active urinary sediments	>1 g proteinuria/day or >0.5 g/day with active urinary sediments	-
Repeat renal biopsy	<50% reduction of proteinuria Worsening GFR Relapse No response to treatment	Worsening GFR No response to treatment or deteriorating renal function	<50% reduction of proteinuria Rising creatinine relapse Worsening disease/no remission after 12 months
Class II LN	Treat extrarenal if proteinuria <1 g/day Cyclosporine/ Azathioprine if proteinuria >1 g/day	-	Treat extrarenal disease If proteinuria >3 g/day, cyclosporine or other calcineurin inhibitors

Class III/IV LN Uniform recommendation of induction with either IV CYC or mycophenolate (doses mentioned only in ACR guideline) and maintenance with azathioprine or mycophenolate

Class V LN—non-nephrotic range proteinuria—treatment for extrarenal disease, for nephrotic range proteinuria cyclophosphamide or mycophenolate (KDIGO prefers MMF over CYC)

Non-responders	Switch immuno-suppressant Alternate—rituximab	Switch immuno-suppressant with pulse methyl prednisolone Alternate—rituximab	Switch immunosuppressant Alternate—rituximab, IVIg
During pregnancy	Low-dose corticosteroid, azathioprine, hydroxy-chloroquine, cyclosporine, low-dose aspirin	Low-dose corticosteroid, azathioprine, hydroxy-chloroquine	Low-dose corticosteroid, azathioprine, hydroxy-chloroquine, low-dose aspirin

pregnancies in lupus patients who are anti-Ro positive and also in mothers with associated antiphospholipid syndrome.

Appropriate doses of vitamin D and calcium are recommended to prevent glucocorticoid induced osteoporosis.

Treatment of APS-associated with SLE is similar to primary APS. Low-dose aspirin is recommended for primary prevention of pregnancy loss, while anticoagulation is recommended for secondary prevention (prophylactic dose of heparin for pregnancy loss and therapeutic doses with past thrombosis). Glucocorticoids, plasma exchange and rituximab are suggested for catastrophic APS.

Rituximab has been recommended by both the ACR and the EULAR guidelines for the treatment of refractory lupus nephritis. Though the two major randomised controlled trials of rituximab (EXPLORER and LUNAR) have failed in lupus, these trials have been criticised for the use of high background medications including corticosteroids and immuno-suppressive. With good results from large prospective studies and registry data, most rheumatologists are comfortable prescribing rituximab primarily for refractory articular, hematologic and renal manifestations of lupus. Experts across the world believe that rituximab can replace steroids in lupus which has paved way to the observational study using the RITUXILUP protocol where mycophenolate and rituximab with no oral steroid led to a complete or partial renal response in 90% at median time of 37 weeks and 86% at 52 weeks.[8]

While belimumab met its primary end point in BLISS-52 and BLISS-76, both the trials excluded active nephritis and neuropsychiatric disease; newer therapies for which are required in lupus. Moreover, its non-availability in India makes it a redundant option as of date. BLISS-LN trial is an ongoing trial to evaluate belimumab in lupus nephritis.

RISKS

The risk of treatment in lupus that every care giver would be worried about are non-response, drug toxicity and non-compliance. With results extrapolated from lupus nephritis trials, it is obvious that about 30% of individuals with lupus do not respond to standard immunosuppression. Despite therapies like belimumab, rituximab, calcineurin inhibitors, IVIg or plasma exchange for refractory disease, about 10–15% of patients still remain non-responders. Except for prednisolone and hydroxychloroquine, it took another 50 years for FDA to approve another drug for lupus in 2011. With the failure of newer therapies like ocrelizumab, veltuzumab (anti-CD 20); Epratuzumab (anti-CD22), abetimus (tolerogen) and anti-interferon therapies, the future seems difficult for lupus.

Several concerns exist regarding the adverse effects of medications used for lupus and with no new medications in the immediate pipeline, clear idea about the dose recommended and the potential adverse effects needs to be known by the treating physician and also communicated appropriately to the patient and their family. Glucocorticoids form the mainstay of therapy in lupus till date with 50–70% patients on GCs at any time point and >90% having received GCs at some time point. No standard dose for GC usage is approved in lupus. While low doses are used for mild lupus, high doses and pulse steroids are used for severe/life-threatening manifestations, with dose being an individualised opinion and no recommendations to guide the same. Data from the Hopkins cohort showed that prednisolone dosages above 6 mg/day increased the risk of future organ damage by 50% and later the same group published data of 2265 patients where prednisolone dose ≥7.5 mg/day had an HR of 1.7 (95% CI 1.5–2.0) to accrue any organ damage compared to <7.5 mg with maximum effect size on cataract, osteoporotic fractures, and cardiovascular damage.[9] Hence, a safer option with least steroid usage has always been and is an ongoing search.

In a network meta-analysis published in 2017, for patients with proliferative lupus nephritis, MMF combined with calcineurin inhibitors was less likely to cause ovarian failure, while the odds of major infection was similar to cyclophosphamide.[10] It is also believed that tacrolimus is a safer option and causes less infections compared to other agents. In a systematic review and network meta-analysis published in February 2018, the same was confirmed. But it was also found that cyclophosphamide or mycophenolate cause lesser number of serious adverse events compared to a combination of mycophenolate and tacrolimus. Gastrointestinal events were least with rituximab, while serious leucopenia was more likely with cyclophosphamide followed by azathioprine and azathioprine alone. Menstrual abnormalities and ovarian failure were highest with cyclophosphamide alone or in combination with any other drug. New onset hypertension was more likely with cyclosporine combined with glucocorticoids. No differences were noted among the immunosuppressive agents, regarding the risk of cardiovascular events, bone toxicity, malignant transformation and hyperglycaemia.[11]

Certain manifestations of lupus either are not addressed or fail to respond to current therapies. Accelerated atherosclerosis and fatigue are two such manifestations. Currently SLE is considered a CAD equivalent and treatment goals for cardiovascular risk factors as in diabetes are recommended but are seldom practised in a routine OPD.[12] Fatigue which is noted in 50–80% of SLE patients has no specific treatment, hinders the quality of life, performance levels and is one of the major reasons for depression. Fatigue being partially a subjective symptom is difficult to assess and hence the lack of adequate research in the same. There is no reliable treatment for fatigue despite most trials measuring fatigue as one of their outcome measures. Addressing sleep disturbances, pain, depression, vitamin D deficiency, maintaining least dose of steroids with a regular paced physical activity have been suggested as the best means to reduce fatigue. Alopecia both due to disease activity and drugs is another challenge to treat and is also one of the main reasons why patients default therapy. Post-inflammatory hyperpigmentation, decrease in appetite, certain neuropsychiatric symptoms are some other manifestations which are also difficult to treat.

Non-compliance is another dread that hovers over the management of lupus. Non-communication by the treating physician, incorrect information, drug toxicity, change in appearance, alluring advertisements by alternate therapies, costs incurred and the variable degree of acceptance by family and friends for long-term treatment are some of the reasons for non-compliance which is one of the most important factors for recurrent flares and long term damage accrual and increased mortality. The negative psychological impact that lifelong disease and its treatment imposes on a patient especially at an age when the family prefers a lady to get married or is just married and is planning a family is a concern that needs addressal.

WHERE LIES THE BALANCE BETWEEN BENEFIT AND RISK IN MANAGEMENT OF LUPUS?

Considering the chronic, relapsing course of lupus with its heterogenous presentation making a uniform study group is difficult and hence the difficulty in conducting large trials in lupus. Besides this, with the exception of lupus nephritis, there is a lack of clear-cut definitions for response assessment in many other important manifestations of lupus.

There have been recent attempts to develop definitions of remission in SLE. The latest definition proposed in 2017, definition of remission in SLE (DORIS) states absent disease in clinical activity [SLEDAI (clinical) = 0 and PGA <0.5 on a scale of 0–3] and organ-based laboratory tests, not including anti-dsDNA antibodies and serum complement. Remission was classified as on therapy and off therapy (on antimalarials alone).[13] A validated definition for low disease activity is LLDAS (lupus low-disease activity state) defined as SLEDAI-2k ≤4, excluding any major organ domains in the SLEDAI or haemolysis and gastrointestinal involvement; no new disease activity; and a physician global assessment (PGA) ≤1 on a scale of 0–3. Treatment was captured in two further domains, requiring a prednisolone (or equivalent) dose of ≤7.5 mg/day and absence of toxic effects of current immunosuppressive treatment. Hence, both disease activity and treatment strategy are being included in these definitions of remission or LDA (low-disease activity) definition in lupus unlike RA.[14]

Unlike in rheumatoid arthritis where the target is the joint, treat to target (T2T) approach in lupus, includes the challenge of multiple organs being the target of therapy However, in 2014, an international task force formulated eleven recommendations as T2T approach in lupus. In summary, remission of organ and systemic manifestations and when not achievable, the lowest the lowest possible disease activity with prevention of flares, minimising damage accrual, improving quality of life by addressing fatigue, pain and depression, controlling comorbidities the lest dose or withdrawal of glucocorticoids were recommended as a realisable treatment target. Use of antimalarials as a part of treatment regimen was recommended, while treatment of clinically inactive serologically active lupus was discouraged. In lupus nephritis, early recognition, induction followed by 3 years of maintenance was recommended. Treatment of antiphospholipid syndrome was recommended.[15]

HOW TO ACHIEVE THE BALANCE?

Maintaining a balance between the benefits of treating a lupus patient and the risks involved is akin to a catch 22 situation. A detailed counselling to the patient, care giver at diagnosis regarding lupus including the nature of disease, improvement in survival over years, efficacy of treatment, expected treatment related adverse events and how to handle bad days and social pressure would be a good start. Counselling sessions as and when required and guiding them on a successful marriage and pregnancy is an additional responsibility of the treating physician in our country where patients look up to us for all major decisions—personal or treatment related. This avoids non-compliance, allows the patient to accept certain adverse events where benefit outweighs the risk and also decreases the chances of fatigue or depression thus improving the overall quality of life.

Avoiding the inadvertent use of medications in lupus is another important way to balance the risk and the benefit. New pragmatic approaches with existing molecules, e.g. combining mycophenolate and calcineurin inhibitors for lupus nephritis and RITUXILUP protocol have shown promising results. Research focussing on newer medications with more efficacy and lesser side effects, research to consider when to withdraw medications without increasing the risk of flare is necessary.

In conclusion, the aim is to have good control of disease activity with minimal toxicity in addition to preventing organ damage and giving a good quality of life to patient. However, it comes at a cost and how to minimize that needs both the art and science of clinical medicine.

REFERENCES

1. Tunnicliffe DJ, Singh-Grewal D, Kim S, Craig JC, Tong A. Diagnosis, monitoring, and treatment of systemic lupus erythematosus: A systematic review of clinical practice guidelines. Arthritis Care Res. 2015 Oct;67(10):1440–52.
2. Bertsias GK, Ioannidis JPA, Aringer M, Bollen E, Bombardieri S, Bruce IN, et al. EULAR recommendations for the management of systemic lupus erythematosus with neuropsychiatric manifestations: Report of a task force of the EULAR standing committee for clinical affairs. Ann Rheum Dis. 2010 Dec;69(12):2074–82.
3. Bertsias G, Ioannidis JPA, Boletis J, Bombardieri S, Cervera R, Dostal C, et al. EULAR recommendations for the management of systemic lupus erythematosus. Report of a task force of the EULAR standing committee for international clinical studies including therapeutics. Ann Rheum Dis. 2008 Feb; 67(2):195–205.
4. Barile-Fabris L, Ariza-Andraca R, Olguín-Ortega L, Jara LJ, Fraga-Mouret A, Miranda-Limón JM, et al. Controlled clinical trial of IV cyclophosphamide versus IV methylprednisolone in severe neurological manifestations in systemic lupus erythematosus. Ann Rheum Dis. 2005 Apr;64(4):620–5.
5. Bertsias GK, Tektonidou M, Amoura Z, Aringer M, Bajema I, Berden JHM, et al. European League Against Rheumatism and European Renal Association-European Dialysis and Transplant Association. Joint European League Against Rheumatism and European Renal Association-European Dialysis and Transplant Association (EULAR/ERA-EDTA) recommendations for the management of adult and paediatric lupus nephritis. Ann Rheum Dis. 2012 Nov;71(11):1771–82.

6. Hahn BH, McMahon MA, Wilkinson A, Wallace WD, Daikh DI, FitzGerald JD, et al. American college of rheumatology guidelines for screening, treatment, and management of lupus nephritis. Arthritis Care Res. 2012 Jun 1;64(6):797–808.

7. Beck L, Bomback AS, Choi MJ, Holzman LB, Langford C, Mariani LH, et al. KDOQI US commentary on the 2012 KDIGO clinical practice guideline for glomerulonephritis. Am J Kidney Dis Off J Natl Kidney Found. 2013 Sep;62(3):403–41.

8. Condor MB, Ashby D, Pepper RJ, Cook HT, Levy JB, Griffith M, et al. Prospective observational single-centre cohort study to evaluate the effectiveness of treating lupus nephritis with rituximab and mycophenolate mofetil but no oral steroids. Ann Rheum Dis. 2013 Aug;72(8):1280–6.

9. Al Sawah S, Zhang X, Zhu B, Magder LS, Foster SA, Iikuni N, et al. Effect of corticosteroid use by dose on the risk of developing organ damage over time in systemic lupus erythematosus-the Hopkins Lupus Cohort. Lupus Sci Med. 2015;2(1):e000066.

10. Palmer SC, Tunnicliffe DJ, Singh-Grewal D, Mavridis D, Tonelli M, Johnson DW, et al. Induction and maintenance immunosuppression treatment of proliferative lupus nephritis: A network meta-analysis of randomized trials. Am J Kidney Dis Off J Natl Kidney Found. 2017 Sep;70(3):324–36.

11. Tian J, Luo Y, Wu H, Long H, Zhao M, Lu Q. Risk of adverse events from different drugs for SLE: A systematic review and network meta-analysis. Lupus Sci Med. 2018;5(1):e000253.

12. Wajed J, Ahmad Y, Durrington PN, Bruce IN. Prevention of cardiovascular disease in systemic lupus erythematosus—proposed guidelines for risk factor management. Rheumatol Oxf Engl. 2004 Jan;43(1):7–12.

13. Van Vollenhoven R, Voskuyl A, Bertsias G, Aranow C, Aringer M, Arnaud L, et al. A framework for remission in SLE: Consensus findings from a large international task force on definitions of remission in SLE (DORIS). Ann Rheum Dis. 2017 Mar;76(3):554–61.

14. Franklyn K, Lau CS, Navarra SV, Louthrenoo W, Lateef A, Hamijoyo L, et al. Definition and initial validation of a lupus low disease activity state (LLDAS). Ann Rheum Dis. 2016 Sep;75(9):1615–21.

15. Van Vollenhoven RF, Mosca M, Bertsias G, Isenberg D, Kuhn A, Lerstrøm K, et al. Treat-to-target in systemic lupus erythematosus: Recommendations from an international task force. Ann Rheum Dis. 2014 Jun;73(6):958–67.

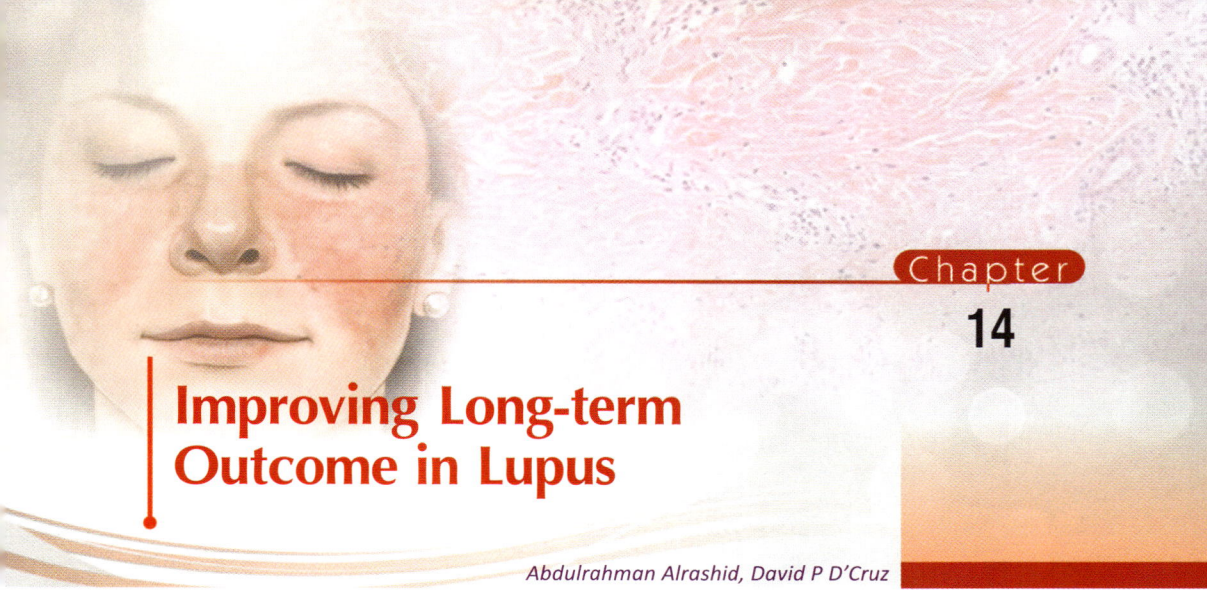

Improving Long-term Outcome in Lupus

Abdulrahman Alrashid, David P D'Cruz

INTRODUCTION

Systemic lupus erythematosus (SLE) is a multi-system autoimmune disease with a wide spectrum of clinical manifestations of varying severity. Previous studies have demonstrated significantly improved 5-year survival rates over the past several decades from 50% to more than 90%. This has been attributed to improvements in diagnostic and classification methods which have led to earlier diagnosis, improved treatment strategies and better control of associated co-morbidities specifically diabetes, hypertension and dyslipidaemia, some of which may be associated with corticosteroid therapy.[1–4] Long-term studies in SLE have demonstrated several poor prognostic factors which can be classified into two categories—modifiable and non-modifiable factors. Non-modifiable factors include age, gender, family history of lupus and ethnicity. These factors may be useful to stratify patients at risk of severe disease and could lead to specific tailored therapies that result in better outcomes.[5–7]

The common causes of mortality in SLE are infection, cardiovascular disease (CVD) and nephritis. Nephritis is a frequent cause of death in developing countries while CVD-related mortality is more prevalent in developed countries.[4,8,9]

This review will focus on the modifiable risk factors with a view to improving the long-term outcome of SLE patients.

EARLY DIAGNOSIS AND PROMPT TREATMENT

The time from the onset of SLE symptoms to diagnosis is critical. Diagnostic delay may result in disease progression with organ involvement and damage accumulation which is known to carry a poor prognosis. Diagnosis of SLE within 6 months of symptom onset is associated with lower disease flare rates and lower health-related costs.[4,10,11] Late diagnosis is associated with organ damage which is a predictor for further damage accumulation.[4,7] Nightingale, et al. showed that the median time from initial lupus symptoms to diagnosis was 26.4 months which reflects a considerable delay in diagnosis and treatment. Achieving early diagnosis of patients in the community is very challenging. Awareness campaigns in the general population and among non-specialist healthcare providers may help in achieving early diagnosis.[11] A major difficulty however is the non-specific nature of symptoms in early disease. Symptoms such as fatigue, arthralgia, hair fall, oral ulcers and intermittent skin rashes may occur in many other medical conditions. Likewise, very early in the disease course anti-nuclear antibody (ANA) testing may be negative or yield very low titres that are not diagnostic. National and international patient support organisations may have a role in raising awareness through publicity campaigns on the internet and social media.

OPTIMIZING IMMUNOSUPPRESSION USAGE AND DISEASE SEVERITY

Once the diagnosis of lupus is established the next step is to assess the burden of disease and organ involvement. The presence of haemolytic anaemia, low complement levels, proteinuria and high SLE disease activity index (SLEDAI) scores more than 10 are associated with poor prognosis and should be managed intensively.[2] The use of corticosteroids is associated with organ damage (cataracts, avascular necrosis and secondary diabetes) and an increased risk of infection.[4,12,13] The risk of infection correlates with higher steroid doses and longer treatment duration.[13]

SLE patients are at risk of pneumocystis pneumonia (PCP) infection which may have a fulminant course. Prophylactic use of trimethoprim-sulfamethoxazole is controversial and not without risk since some SLE patients are allergic to the sulphur component of this combination. There is therefore no consensus about usage of long-term prophylactic antibiotic in SLE patients. However, this decision should be individualized based on a benefit-risk ratio assessment for a given patient.[13,14]

The cornerstone of management after assessing disease severity is to use the minimum dose of corticosteroids and immunosuppression to control the disease and aiming to minimize the risk of medication side effects. In brief, avoid overtreatment or undertreatment.[15]

VACCINATION IN SLE

Patients with systemic lupus erythematosus are at increased risk of infection either because of the immune system dysregulation caused by lupus itself or from the use of immuno-suppressive medications. Influenza and pneumococcal infections in patients with SLE are associated with significant morbidities and mortality. Influenza and pneumococcal vaccines are effective and safe methods to reduce these risks especially prior to commencing potent immunosuppression including with biologic agents such as rituximab and belimumab.[16–19]

Vaccination is therefore an important strategy to reduce the rate of infection. Studies showed that most vaccines are effective and safe in lupus patients. As a rule, live-attenuated vaccines should be avoided in all immunocompromised patients.[13,16,20] This advice may change in the future. The effects of some vaccines may be attenuated in patients already on immunosuppressive therapies especially biologics such as rituximab, so ideally patients should be vaccinated prior to starting these therapies.

The European League against Rheumatism (EULAR) guidelines recommend hepatitis B vaccination in SLE patients with increased risk of infection for example living in or travel to endemic countries and working in the health care professions or living with an infected family member.[16,21]

REGULAR CLINICAL AND LABORATORY FOLLOW-UP

The primary aim in the management of SLE patients is to achieve remission or low disease activity. Lupus patients are at risk of developing disease flares with associated co-morbidities and medication adverse effects. Accordingly, regular close clinical follow up and disease activity assessments are recommended and form a part of international guidelines. History taking, complete physical examination and laboratory work up should be carried out at each clinical visit to detect early disease flares and monitor for treatment toxicities.[15,22–24]

All lupus patients should be managed by specialist rheumatologists to achieve better outcomes with minimum cost.[25] Long-term follow-up assessments are recommended for non-active lupus with no organ damage every 6–12 months. For patients with mild disease assessments every 3–6 months are recommended. Closer follow up is required for patients with severe disease and prior to pregnancy, organ transplant or surgery.[23]

Prevention of Disease Flares

More than half of patients with SLE may experience disease flares after a period of disease control. Studies clearly showed that recurrent disease flares are associated with organ damage accumulation and poor outcomes.[7,15,26–28]

The treat-to-target in systemic lupus erythematosus task force conclude that "flare prevention should be a therapeutic goal, and that it is a realistic target".[15]

Predictors of clinical lupus flares include past lupus nephritis, neurological manifestations,[27] vasculitis, elevated anti-dsDNA or B lymphocyte stimulator levels, or low C3. Close follow up and monitoring of patients with these risk factors may help in the prevention or detection of early clinical flare ups.[29] Patients should also be counselled on how to recognise symptoms of disease flares and clinics should make access easy for flaring patients depending on resource availability.

AVOIDING ULTRA-VIOLET RADIATION

Multiple environmental exposures were identified as trigger factors for lupus flares. Ultra-violet (UV) radiation is one of these factors that can provoke photosensitivity. Many studies have demonstrated that SLE flares are more common during summer and are linked to direct sun exposure.[30–32]

Patient education about the association between disease flares and UV exposure is important. All patients with SLE and a history of photosensitivity should consider using photoprotective measures. The use of broad-spectrum sunscreens and in some cases photoprotective clothing have a role in preventing photosensitivity and minimising the risk of generalised disease flares following exposure to UV radiation.[30,31,33,34] Less renal involvement, thrombocytopenia and hospitalization were observed in patients with SLE using sunscreen.[35]

ROLE OF HYDROXYCHLOROQUINE (HCQ)

HCQ is well tolerated, has a good safety profile and established therapeutic and prophylactic effects against lupus flares. It should be considered in all patients with SLE (even during pregnancy) unless contraindicated.[15,25,36–41]

HCQ has a favourable effect in reducing flares,[15,36] decreasing damage accumulation,[15] improving skin manifestations and survival.[15,36,39–41] Moreover, it has a protective effect against Metabolic syndrome[42] and thrombosis[43] in SLE patients.

HCQ use in lupus is associated with valuable protective effects in the short and long term. Data also supports HCQ use not only in protecting against mild-moderate flares but major flares too.[37,38]

A study of more than 2300 patients using HCQ showed the overall prevalence of hydroxychloroquine retinopathy was 7.5%.[44] In February 2018, the UK Royal College of Ophthalmologists Clinical Guidelines for hydroxychloroquine and chloroquine retinopathy Screening recommended a baseline eye examination within the first year of starting HCQ, then after 5 years of taking the medication and annually thereafter by an ophthalmologist.[45] Accordingly, all patients using HCQ should be referred for a retinal screening program.

NON-ADHERENCE TO MEDICATION

One of the commonest causes of disease flares and poor outcomes is non-adherence to prescribed medication and failure to attend clinic appointments. This phenomenon is seen in all branches of medicine and is not specific to patients with rheumatic diseases. Measuring medication non-adherence is notoriously difficult as patients frequently do not admit to non-adherence. Non-adherence may be intentional or more commonly non-intentional. Intentional non-adherence, where the patient never actually starts taking the medication, may have many causes. These include complex medication regimens, failure to understand the reasons for therapies, lack of educational attainment, lack of trust in the healthcare provider and language and cultural barriers among others. Non-intentional non-adherence may be due to forgetting to renew prescriptions, losing medications and forgetting to take individual doses.

Measuring drug levels such as hydroxychloroquine and mycophenolate levels can estimate the level of non-adherence, but these can be confounded by patients taking medications just before a clinic visit.[46]

A particularly concerning study from the USA showed that in patients with SLE in the Medicaid program, only 17% of patients starting azathioprine and 21% of patients starting mycophenolate mofetil were adherent.[47] This was similar to a previous study that showed that in Medicaid patients initiating hydroxychloroquine, only 17% were persistent adherers and 36% were persistent non-adherers. Furthermore, adherence declined for most patients over the first year.[48]

Improving medication adherence remains very challenging due to the complexity of the problem and lack of awareness among healthcare providers of the scale of the problem.

METABOLIC SYNDROME AND LIFESTYLE MEASURES

Non-pharmacological interventions are important in improving disease control and recent attention has focused on clinical trials. In 2008, the EULAR recommended positive lifestyle changes in the management of lupus which include physical activity, weight control and smoking cessation.[22]

Metabolic Syndrome

The metabolic syndrome is the constellation of central obesity, dyslipidaemia, hypertension and disturbed glucose metabolism.[49] These factors are associated with significant morbidities (organ damage and cardiovascular events) and mortality in patients with SLE.[22,42,50–52] Specifically, smoking and hypertension are risk factors for renal failure in SLE.[53] In SLE patients with metabolic syndrome, higher levels of inflammatory markers were observed.[54]

The presence of metabolic syndrome in SLE should be addressed carefully as it may worsen the cumulative organ damage and enhance the adverse effects of medications such as corticosteroids and calcineurin inhibitors (CNIs).[23] Risk factors for developing metabolic syndrome include recent disease activity, the duration of high dose corticosteroid exposure and depression. Antimalarial drugs should be considered to reduce the risk of development of the metabolic syndrome.[55]

Renin-angiotensin system blockade by angiotensin-converting enzyme (ACE) inhibitors or angiotensin receptor blockers (ARB) is the cornerstone in the management of high blood pressure, controlling proteinuria and have a renal protective benefit in SLE patients with nephritis.[56,57]

Statin use to control lipids is associated with significant reductions in morbidities and mortality.[54,58,59]

Disease activity control by using antimalarial drugs and rituximab can help in improving lipid profiles supporting the notion that autoimmune disease can provoke dyslipidaemia.[42,60] By contrast, corticosteroid use may exacerbate dyslipidemia and increases the risk of the metabolic syndrome and should be minimised wherever possible. The usual standard approach to prednisolone dosing of 1 mg/kg/day is not evidence based and is nearly always excessive and times prednisolone taper should be rapid with use of steroid sparing agents.

Estimating the risk of CVD and taking a prompt measure to eliminate or reduce the risk are a practical strategy. There are several cardiovascular disease risk calculators and the QRISK3 algorithm recently incorporated SLE as an additional risk factor for CVD. This model should be used in all SLE patients to stratify CVD risk and guide interventions to improve outcomes.[61,62]

Diet and Weight Loss

SLE outcomes can be improved by optimizing diet and lifestyle measures. SLE patients are at risk of metabolic syndrome, anaemia and low-bone density.[54,63,64]

Recent studies demonstrated the beneficial effects of a Mediterranean type diet on the risk of cancer, high blood pressure, lipid profile, insulin resistance and has an anti-inflammatory effect. This diet is rich in olive oil, plant foods (fruits, vegetables, cereals, nuts and seeds, moderate consumption of fish, seafood, yogurt, cheese, poultry and eggs and low red meat intake).[65,66] There is beneficial evidence of mono- and polyunsaturated fatty acids as it has anti-inflammatory and cardiovascular protective effects.[67] SLE patients should therefore be encouraged to eat a healthy diet, especially as one study showed that these patients had inadequate nutritional intake.[68]

Lupus patients with obesity are different from lupus patients with normal weight, as they may have higher damage scores, cholesterol levels, blood sugar and high blood pressure.[69] Measures to achieve the ideal body weight should be considered in all patients.

There is evidence that losing weight in lupus patients is associated with decreased immunosuppression dosage. Only one trial studied the outcome of bariatric surgery in SLE patients which showed that the overall risk is higher than the general population, but the benefit was clear. This surgical intervention should be considered carefully with an evaluation of the benefits and risks.[70]

Exercise

Exercise is safe and has a favourable effect in lupus by improving aerobic fitness, fatigue and depression.[71–73] Exercise could have synergetic anti-inflammatory effects and minimize medication adverse effects such as low bone or muscle mass, metabolic syndrome and low immunity.[72]

There is no consensus about a specific exercise program in SLE patients.

Smoking Cessation

Smoking has a negative impact on overall health. Studies showed higher damage scores in African–American SLE patients compared to other ethnicities and smoking and sedentary lifestyle were more prevalent in this group.[74] Smoking cessation should be considered by the treating clinician, but it is unfortunately frequently ignored in clinical practice.[50,75]

Smoking is associated with poor outcomes in lupus with greater organ damage and more disease activity.[76,77] Impaired antimalarial effects were observed in smokers with refractory cutaneous disease.[78,79] Moreover, smoking is a risk factor for thrombosis[43] and renal failure[53] in SLE patients.

Education to enhance smoking cessation in lupus patients should be considered.

HUMAN PAPILLOMAVIRUS (HPV) AND SLE

Human Papillomavirus (HPV) infections are common in SLE patients which can lead to cervical dysplasia. Previous studies showed a 9-fold increased risk in pre-malignant cervical lesions in lupus patients compared with healthy populations. This warrants consideration of cervical cancer screening and HPV vaccination in lupus patients.[16,21,80,81]

The EULAR recommendations state that HPV vaccine should be considered in patients with autoimmune inflammatory rheumatic diseases.[21]

BONE HEALTH AND SLE

The musculoskeletal system is commonly involved in SLE. Osteoporosis and avascular necrosis are frequent bone health issues in rheumatology clinics with a high burden affecting patients' quality of life with high healthcare costs.[82] Glucocorticoids disease activity and cumulative organ damage are established risk factors for osteoporosis in SLE.[82–84] All SLE patients should receive calcium and vitamin D supplementation while on long-term glucocorticoids as bone protection.[22,24,82]

Dual-energy X-ray absorptiometry (DEXA) scanning is the most useful tool for diagnosing and monitoring bone density. All patients on long-term glucocorticoids should have a DEXA scan at baseline then every 3–5 years depending on the presence of other risk factors.[24] The fracture risk assessment (FRAX) tool is a calculator of fracture likelihood, although steroid dose or duration are not considered in the FRAX calculation. Accordingly, it might underestimate fracture risk in SLE patients.[82] It has a benefit over the DEXA scan as its calculation does not need any equipment. The Canadian Rheumatology Association recommends it as a screening tool for osteoporosis in SLE patients.[85]

Bisphosphonates are the main treatment for osteoporosis. Since the bone loss is higher initially with steroid use, bisphosphonates should be considered concurrently with long-term steroid use especially in high risk groups, although this is uncommon in clinical practice.[84,86] A meta-analysis of bisphosphonate use in SLE showed improvements in bone mineral density and lower fracture rates.[87]

Teriparatide is a human recombinant parathyroid hormone that showed superiority to bisphosphonates in terms of improving bone density and reducing fracture rates in glucocorticoid-induced osteoporosis in SLE.[88,89]

Denosumab is a monoclonal antibody approved for primary osteoporosis treatment. Studies have showed beneficial effects in improving bone density and lower fracture rates in osteoporosis secondary to steroid use.[90,91]

Avascular bone necrosis (AVN) is another serious bone health-related issue in SLE patients. A large cohort study showed the prevalence of symptomatic AVN was 13.6%.[92] All patients with suggestive pain related to AVN should undergo plain radiography, and if not diagnostic, magnetic resonance imaging (MRI) should be considered.[23,85]

Glucocorticoid use and high disease activity are strong risk factors for AVN. Other predictive factors are the use of cytotoxic drugs, arthritis, renal disease and neuropsychiatric manifestations of SLE.[92–97]

All measures to control disease activity and minimise glucocorticoid doses should be considered to protect the bone and avoid these serious complications. Earlier introduction of steroid sparing agents will help to avoid glucocorticoid adverse effects.

PATIENT EDUCATION AND SOCIAL SUPPORT

Considering social aspects in managing lupus is critical as poor social support and socioeconomic status are clearly associated with negative outcomes of lupus.[12,98] In one study, annual family income less than $25,000 impacted negatively on lupus survival.[2] SLE has a huge burden on quality of life and financial status. Most patients reported less socializing and significant impact on their employment after SLE was diagnosed.[99]

Disease awareness campaign in the community, social media and among employers should lead to better social support and disease outcomes.

CONCLUSION

While there is no doubt that the outlook for patients with SLE has improved enormously over the last 50 years, there are still challenges in improving morbidity, mortality and quality of life. Efforts to improve patient outcomes should start with early diagnosis and continue throughout the patients' lifetime. This should clearly be a multidisciplinary effort involving the patient and their family wherever possible.

REFERENCES

1. Uramoto KM, Jr. CJM, Thumboo J, Sunku J, Ofallon WM, Gabriel SE. Trends in the incidence and mortality of systemic lupus erythematosus, 1950–1992. Arthritis and Rheumatism. 1999;42(1):46–50.
2. Kasitanon N, Magder LS, Petri M. Predictors of survival in systemic lupus erythematosus. Medicine. 2006;85(3):147–56.
3. Doria A, Iaccarino L, Ghirardello A, Zampieri S, Arienti S, Sarzi-Puttini P, et al. Long-term prognosis and causes of death in systemic lupus erythematosus. Am J Med. 2006; 119(8):700–6.
4. Mok CC, Mak A, Chu WP, To CH, Wong SN. Long-term survival of Southern Chinese patients with systemic lupus erythematosus. Medicine. 2005;84(4):218–24.
5. Bruce IN, Okeeffe AG, Farewell V, Hanly JG, Manzi S, Su L, et al. Factors associated with damage accrual in patients with systemic lupus erythematosus: Results from the systemic lupus international collaborating clinics (SLICC) inception cohort. Ann Rheum Dis. 2014;74(9):1706–13.
6. Gómez-Puerta JA, Barbhaiya M, Guan H, Feldman CH, Alarcón GS, Costenbader KH. Racial/ethnic variation in all-cause mortality among United States Medicaid recipients with systemic lupus erythematosus: A hispanic and Asian paradox. Arthritis Rheumatol. 2015;67(3):752–60.
7. Bruce IN, Okeeffe AG, Farewell V, Hanly JG, Manzi S, Su L, et al. Factors associated with damage accrual in patients with systemic lupus erythematosus: results from the systemic lupus international collaborating clinics (SLICC) inception cohort. Ann Rheum Dis. 2014;74(9):1706–13.

8. Cervera R, Khamashta MA, Font J, Sebastiani GD, Gil A, Lavilla P, et al. Morbidity and mortality in systemic lupus erythematosus during a 10-year period. Medicine. 2003;82(5):299–308.

9. Souza DC, Santo AH, Sato EI. Mortality profile related to systemic lupus erythematosus: A multiple cause-of-death analysis. J Rheumatol. 2012;39(3):496–503.

10. Oglesby A, Dennis G, Korves C, Laliberté F, Suthoff E, Wei R, et al. PSY56 impact of early versus late systemic lupus erythematosus (SLE) diagnosis on clinical and economic outcomes. Value in Health. 2012;15(4).

11. Nightingale AL, Davidson JE, Molta CT, Kan HJ, Mchugh NJ. Presentation of SLE in UK primary care using the clinical practice research datalink. Lupus Sci Med. 2017;4(1).

12. Ward MM. Education level and mortality in systemic lupus erythematosus (SLE): Evidence of underascertainment of deaths due to SLE in ethnic minorities with low education levels. Arthritis Care Res. 2004;51(4):616–24.

13. Falagas ME, Manta KG, Betsi GI, Pappas G. Infection-related morbidity and mortality in patients with connective tissue diseases: A systematic review. Clin Rheumatol. 2006;26(5):663–70.

14. Kronbichler A, Kerschbaum J, Gopaluni S, Tieu J, Alberici F, Jones RB, et al. Trimethoprim-sulfamethoxazole prophylaxis prevents severe/life-threatening infections following rituximab in antineutrophil cytoplasm antibody-associated vasculitis. Ann Rheum Dis. 2018;77(10):1440–47.

15. Vollenhoven RFV, Mosca M, Bertsias G, Isenberg D, Kuhn A, Lerstrøm K, et al. Treat-to-target in systemic lupus erythematosus: Recommendations from an international task force. Ann Rheum Dis. 2014;73(6):958–67.

16. Garg M, Mufti N, Palmore TN, Hasni SA. Recommendations and barriers to vaccination in systemic lupus erythematosus. Autoimmunity Reviews. 2018;17(10):990–1001.

17. Grabar S, Groh M, Bahuaud M, Guern VL, Costedoat-Chalumeau N, Mathian A, et al. Pneumococcal vaccination in patients with systemic lupus erythematosus: A multicenter placebo-controlled randomized double-blind study. Vaccine. 2017;35(37):4877–85.

18. Mcfetridge R, Meulen AS-T, Folkerth SD, Hoekstra JA, Dallas M, Hoover PA, et al. Safety, tolerability, and immunogenicity of 15-valent pneumococcal conjugate vaccine in healthy adults. Vaccine. 2015;33(24):2793–9.

19. Chang C-C, Chang Y-S, Chen W-S, Chen Y-H, Chen J-H. Effects of annual influenza vaccination on morbidty and mortality in patients with systemic lupus erythematosus: A nationwide cohort study. Scientific Reports. 2016;6(1).

20. Grein IHR, Groot N, Lacerda MI, Wulffraat N, Pileggi G. HPV infection and vaccination in Systemic Lupus Erythematosus patients: What we really should know. Ped Rheumatol. 2016;14(1).

21. Assen SV, Agmon-Levin N, Elkayam O, Cervera R, Doran MF, Dougados M, et al. EULAR recommendations for vaccination in adult patients with autoimmune inflammatory rheumatic diseases. Ann Rheum Dis. 2010;70(3):414–22.

22. Bertsias G, Ioannidis J, Boletis J, Bombardieri S, Cervera R, Dostal C, et al. New EULAR guidelines about treatment systemic lupus eritematosus. Rheumatol Sci Pract. 2008;(1):93.

23. Guidelines for referral and management of systemic lupus erythematosus in adults. Arthritis Rheumat. 1999;42(9):1785–96.

24. Tunnicliffe DJ, Singh-Grewal D, Kim S, Craig JC, Tong A. Diagnosis, monitoring, and treatment of systemic lupus erythematosus: A systematic review of clinical practice guidelines. Arthritis Care Res. 2015;67(10):1440–52.

25. Kan H, Nagar S, Patel J, Wallace DJ, Molta C, Chang DJ. Longitudinal treatment patterns and associated outcomes in patients with newly diagnosed systemic lupus erythematosus. Clin Ther. 2016;38(3):610–24.

26. Stoll T. Analysis of the relationship between disease activity and damage in patients with systemic lupus erythematosus—a 5-yr prospective study. Rheumatology. 2004;43(8):1039–44.

27. Mak A, Cheung MW-L, Chiew HJ, Liu Y, Ho RC-M. Global trend of survival and damage of systemic lupus erythematosus: Meta-analysis and meta-regression of observational studies from the 1950s to 2000s. Sem Arthritis Rheum. 2012;41(6):830–9.

28. Sutton EJ, Davidson JE, Bruce IN. The systemic lupus international collaborating clinics (SLICC) damage index: A systematic literature review. Sem Arthritis Rheum. 2013;43(3):352–61.

29. Petri MA, Vollenhoven RFV, Buyon J, Levy RA, Navarra SV, Cervera R, et al. Baseline predictors of systemic lupus erythematosus flares: Data from the combined placebo groups in the phase III Belimumab Trials. Arthritis Rheum. 2013;65(8):2143–53.

30. Barbhaiya M, Costenbader K. Ultraviolet radiation and systemic lupus erythematosus. Lupus. 2014; 23(6):588–95.

31. Kuhn A, Beissert S. Photosensitivity in lupus erythematosus. Autoimmunity. 2005;38(7):519–29.

32. Cooper GS, Wither J, Bernatsky S, Claudio JO, Clarke A, Rioux JD, et al. Occupational and environmental exposures and risk of systemic lupus erythematosus: Silica, sunlight, solvents. Rheumatology. 2010;49(11):2172–80.

33. Kuhn A, Gensch K, Haust M, Meuth A-M, Boyer F, Dupuy P, et al. Photoprotective effects of a broad-spectrum sunscreen in ultraviolet-induced cutaneous lupus erythematosus: A randomized, vehicle-controlled, double-blind study. J Am Acad Dermatol. 2011;64(1):37–48.

34. Stege H, Budde M-A, Grether-Beck S, Krutmann J. Evaluation of the capacity of sunscreens to photoprotect lupus erythematosus patients by employing the photoprovocation test. Photodermatology, Photoimmunology and Photomedicine. 2000;16(6):256–9.

35. Vilá LM, Mayor AM, Valentín AH, Rodríguez SI, Reyes ML, Acosta E, et al. Association of sunlight exposure and photoprotection measures with clinical outcome in systemic lupus erythematosus. P R Health Sci J. 1999 Jun;18(2):89–94.

36. Ugarte-Gil MF, Wojdyla D, Pastor-Asurza CA, Gamboa-Cárdenas RV, Acevedo-Vásquez EM, Catoggio LJ, et al. Predictive factors of flares in systemic lupus erythematosus patients: Data from a multiethnic Latin American cohort. Lupus. 2017;27(4):536–44.

37. The Canadain Hydroxychloroquine Study Group. A randomized study of the effect of withdrawing hydroxychloroquine sulfate in systemic lupus erythematosus. New Engl J Med. 1991;324(3):150–4.

38. Tsakonas E, Joseph L, Esdaile JM, Choquette D, Senécal J-L, Cividino A, et al. A Long-term study of hydroxychloroquine withdrawal on exacerbations in systemic lupus erythematosus. Lupus. 1998; 7(2):80–5.

39. Ruiz-Irastorza G, Ramos-Casals M, Brito-Zeron P, Khamashta MA. Clinical efficacy and side effects of antimalarials in systemic lupus erythematosus: A systematic review. Ann Rheum DIs. 2008;69(01):20–8.

40. Shinjo SK, Bonfá E, Wojdyla D, Borba EF, Ramirez LA, Scherbarth HR, et al. Antimalarial treatment may have a time-dependent effect on lupus survival: Data from a multinational Latin American inception cohort. Arthritis Rheum. 2010;62(3):855–62.

41. Alarcon GS, Mcgwin G, Bertoli AM, Fessler BJ, Calvo-Alen J, Bastian HM, et al. Effect of hydroxychloroquine on the survival of patients with systemic lupus erythematosus: data from LUMINA, a multiethnic US cohort (LUMINA L). Ann Rheum Dis. 2007;66(9):1168–72.

42. Mok CC, Tse SM, Chan KL, Ho LY. Effect of the metabolic syndrome on organ damage and mortality in patients with systemic lupus erythematosus: A longitudinal analysis. Clin Exp Rheumatol. 2018 May-Jun;36(3):389–95.

43. Kaiser R, Cleveland CM, Criswell LA. Risk and protective factors for thrombosis in systemic lupus erythematosus: Results from a large, multi-ethnic cohort. Ann Rheum Dis. 2009 Feb;68(2):238–41.

44. Melles RB, Marmor MF. The risk of toxic retinopathy in patients on long-term hydroxychloroquine therapy. JAMA Ophthalmol. 2014 Dec;132(12):1453–60.

45. The Royal College of Ophthalmologist. Hydroxychloroquine and chloroquine retinopathy: Recommendations on screening. February 2018.

46. Costedoat-Chalumeau N, Houssiau F, Izmirly P, Guern V, Navarra S, Jolly M, et al. A prospective international study on adherence to treatment in 305 patients with flaring SLE: Assessment by drug levels and self-administered questionnaires. Clin Pharmacol Ther. 2019 Aug;106(2):374–82.

47. Feldman CH, Collins J, Zhang Z, Xu C, Subramanian S, Kawachi I, et al. Azathioprine and mycophenolate mofetil adherence patterns and predictors among medicaid beneficiaries with systemic lupus erythematosus. Arthritis Care Res (Hoboken). 2019 Nov;71(11):1419–24.

48. Feldman CH, Collins J, Zhang Z, Subramanian SV, Solomon DH, Kawachi I, et al. Dynamic patterns and predictors of hydroxychloroquine nonadherence among Medicaid beneficiaries with systemic lupus erythematosus. Semin Arthritis Rheum. 2018;48(2):205–13.

49. Ford ES, Giles WH, Dietz WH. Prevalence of the metabolic syndrome among US adults: Findings from the third National Health and Nutrition Examination Survey. JAMA. 2002 Jan 16;287(3):356–9.
50. Trager J, Ward MM. Mortality and causes of death in systemic lupus erythematosus. Curr Opin Rheumatol. 2001;13(5):345–51.
51. Aviña-Zubieta JA, To F, Vostretsova K, De Vera M, Sayre EC, Esdaile JM. Risk of myocardial infarction and stroke in newly diagnosed systemic lupus erythematosus: A general population-based study. Arthritis Care Res (Hoboken). 2017 06;69(6):849–56.
52. Lilleby V, Flatø B, Førre O. Disease duration, hypertension and medication requirements are associated with organ damage in childhood-onset systemic lupus erythematosus. Clin Exp Rheumatol. 2005 Mar–Apr;23(2):261–9.
53. Ward MM, Studenski S. Clinical prognostic factors in lupus nephritis. The importance of hypertension and smoking. Arch Intern Med. 1992 Oct;152(10):2082–8.
54. Chung CP, Avalos I, Oeser A, Gebretsadik T, Shintani A, Raggi P, et al. High prevalence of the metabolic syndrome in patients with systemic lupus erythematosus: Association with disease characteristics and cardiovascular risk factors. Ann Rheum Dis. 2007 Feb;66(2):208–14.
55. Margiotta DPE, Basta F, Dolcini G, Batani V, Navarini L, Afeltra A. The relation between, metabolic syndrome and quality of life in patients with systemic lupus erythematosus. PLoS ONE. 2017;12(11): e0187645.
56. Yue C, Li G, Wen Y, Li X, Gao R. Early renin-angiotensin system blockade improved short-term and long-term renal outcomes in systemic lupus erythematosus patients with antiphospholipid-associated Nephropathy. J Rheumatol. 2018 May;45(5):655–62.
57. Durán-Barragán S, McGwin G, Vilá LM, Reveille JD, Alarcón GS. Angiotensin-converting enzyme inhibitors delay the occurrence of renal involvement and are associated with a decreased risk of disease activity in patients with systemic lupus erythematosus—results from LUMINA (LIX): a multiethnic US cohort. Rheumatology (Oxford). 2008 Jul;47(7):1093–6.
58. Orge AM, Lu N, Keller SF, Rai SK, Zhang Y, Choi HK. The effect of statin use on mortality in systemic autoimmune rheumatic diseases. J Rheumatol. 2018 Dec;45(12):1689–95.
59. Yu HH, Chen PC, Yang YH, Wang LC, Lee JH, Lin YT, et al. Statin reduces mortality and morbidity in systemic lupus erythematosus patients with hyperlipidemia: A nationwide population-based cohort study. Atherosclerosis. 2015 Nov;243(1):11–8.
60. Pego-Reigosa JM, Lu TY, Fontanillo MF, del Campo-Pérez V, Rahman A, Isenberg DA. Long-term improvement of lipid profile in patients with refractory systemic lupus erythematosus treated with B-cell depletion therapy: A retrospective observational study. Rheumatology (Oxford). 2010 Apr;49(4): 691–6.
61. Hippisley-Cox J, Coupland C, Brindle P. Development and validation of QRISK3 risk prediction algorithms to estimate future risk of cardiovascular disease: Prospective cohort study. BMJ. 2017 May 23;357:j2099.
62. Edwards N, Langford-Smith AWW, Parker BJ, Bruce IN, Reynolds JA, Alexander MY, et al. QRISK3 improves detection of cardiovascular disease risk in patients with systemic lupus erythematosus. Lupus Sci Med. 2018;5(1):e000272.
63. Shah M, Adams-Huet B, Kavanaugh A, Coyle Y, Lipsky P. Nutrient intake and diet quality in patients with systemic lupus erythematosus on a culturally sensitive cholesterol lowering dietary program. J Rheumatol. 2004 Jan;31(1):71–5.
64. Bruce IN. 'Not only...but also': factors that contribute to accelerated atherosclerosis and premature coronary heart disease in systemic lupus erythematosus. Rheumatology (Oxford). 2005 Dec; 44(12):1492–502.
65. Toledo E, Hu FB, Estruch R, Buil-Cosiales P, Corella D, Salas-Salvadó J, et al. Effect of the Mediterranean diet on blood pressure in the PREDIMED trial: Results from a randomized controlled trial. BMC Med. 2013 Sep 19;11:207.
66. Casas R, Sacanella E, Estruch R. The immune protective effect of the Mediterranean diet against chronic low-grade inflammatory diseases. EndocrMetab Immune Disord Drug Targets. 2014;14(4): 245–54.

67. Klack K, Bonfa E, BorbaNeto EF. Diet and nutritional aspects in systemic lupus erythematosus. Rev Bras Reumatol. 2012 May–Jun;52(3):384–408.

68. Borges MC, dos Santos Fde M, Telles RW, Lanna CC, Correia MI. Nutritional status and food intake in patients with systemic lupus erythematosus. Nutrition. 2012 Nov–Dec;28(11–12):1098–103.

69. Moura dos Santos Fde M, Borges MC, Telles RW, Correia MI, Lanna CC. Excess weight and associated risk factors in patients with systemic lupus erythematosus. Rheumatol Int. 2013 Mar;33(3):681–8.

70. Corcelles R, Daigle CR, Talamas HR, Batayyah E, Brethauer SA, Schauer PR. Bariatric surgery outcomes in patients with systemic lupus erythematosus. Surg Obes Relat Dis. 2015 May-Jun;11(3):684–8.

71. O'Dwyer T, Durcan L, Wilson F. Exercise and physical activity in systemic lupus erythematosus: A systematic review with meta-analyses. Semin Arthritis Rheum. 2017 10;47(2):204–15.

72. Perandini LA, de Sá-Pinto AL, Roschel H, Benatti FB, Lima FR, Bonfá E, et al. Exercise as a therapeutic tool to counteract inflammation and clinical symptoms in autoimmune rheumatic diseases. Autoimmun Rev. 2012 Dec;12(2):218–24.

73. Wu ML, Yu KH, Tsai JC. The effectiveness of exercise in adults with systemic lupus erythematosus: A systematic review and meta-analysis to guide evidence-based practice. Worldviews Evid Based Nurs. 2017 Aug;14(4):306–15.

74. Borchers AT, Keen CL, Shoenfeld Y, Gershwin ME. Surviving the butterfly and the wolf: Mortality trends in systemic lupus erythematosus. Autoimmun Rev. 2004 Aug;3(6):423–53.

75. Bruce IN, Gladman DD, Urowitz MB. Detection and modification of risk factors for coronary artery disease in patients with systemic lupus erythematosus: A quality improvement study. Clin Exp Rheumatol. 1998 Jul–Aug;16(4):435–40.

76. Montes RA, Mocarzel LO, Lanzieri PG, Lopes LM, Carvalho A, Almeida JR. Smoking and its association with morbidity in systemic lupus erythematosus evaluated by the systemic lupus international collaborating clinics/American college of rheumatology damage index: Preliminary data and systematic review. Arthritis Rheumatol. 2016;68(2):441–8.

77. Ghaussy NO, Sibbitt W, Bankhurst AD, Qualls CR. Cigarette smoking and disease activity in systemic lupus erythematosus. J Rheumatol. 2003 Jun;30(6):1215–21.

78. Chasset F, Francès C, Barete S, Amoura Z, Arnaud L. Influence of smoking on the efficacy of antimalarials in cutaneous lupus: A meta-analysis of the literature. J Am Acad Dermatol. 2015 Apr; 72(4):634–9.

79. Ezra N, Jorizzo J. Hydroxychloroquine and smoking in patients with cutaneous lupus erythematosus. Clin Exp Dermatol. 2012 Jun;37(4):327–34.

80. Santana IU, Gomes Ado N, Lyrio LD, Rios Grassi MF, Santiago MB. Systemic lupus erythematosus, human papillomavirus infection, cervical pre-malignant and malignant lesions: A systematic review. Clin Rheumatol. 2011 May;30(5):665–72.

81. Zard E, Arnaud L, Mathian A, Chakhtoura Z, Hie M, Touraine P, et al. Increased risk of high grade cervical squamous intraepithelial lesions in systemic lupus erythematosus: A meta-analysis of the literature. Autoimmun Rev. 2014 Jul;13(7):730–5.

82. Edens C, Robinson AB. Systemic lupus erythematosus, bone health, and osteoporosis. Curr Opin Endocrinol Diabetes Obes. 2015 Dec;22(6):422–31.

83. Zhu TY, Griffith JF, Au SK, Tang XL, Kwok AW, Leung PC, et al. Bone mineral density change in systemic lupus erythematosus: A 5-year followup study. J Rheumatol. 2014 Oct;41(10):1990–7.

84. Gilboe IM, Kvien TK, Haugeberg G, Husby G. Bone mineral density in systemic lupus erythematosus: comparison with rheumatoid arthritis and healthy controls. Ann Rheum Dis. 2000 Feb;59(2):110–5.

85. Keeling SO, Alabdurubalnabi Z, Avina-Zubieta A, Barr S, Bergeron L, Bernatsky S, et al. Canadian rheumatology association recommendations for the assessment and monitoring of systemic lupus erythematosus. J Rheumatol. 2018 Oct;45(10):1426–39.

86. Klop C, de Vries F, Vinks T, Kooij MJ, van Staa TP, Bijlsma JW, et al. Increase in prophylaxis of glucocorticoid-induced osteoporosis by pharmacist feedback: A randomised controlled trial. Osteoporos Int. 2014 Jan;25(1):385–92.

87. Feng Z, Zeng S, Wang Y, Zheng Z, Chen Z. Bisphosphonates for the prevention and treatment of osteoporosis in patients with rheumatic diseases: A systematic review and meta-analysis. PLoS ONE. 2013;8(12):e80890.
88. Glüer CC, Marin F, Ringe JD, Hawkins F, Möricke R, Papaioannu N, et al. Comparative effects of teriparatide and risedronate in glucocorticoid-induced osteoporosis in men: 18-month results of the EuroGIOPs trial. J Bone Miner Res. 2013 Jun;28(6):1355–68.
89. Saag KG, Zanchetta JR, Devogelaer JP, Adler RA, Eastell R, See K, et al. Effects of teriparatide versus alendronate for treating glucocorticoid-induced osteoporosis: Thirty-six-month results of a randomized, double-blind, controlled trial. Arthritis Rheum. 2009 Nov;60(11):3346–55.
90. Dore RK, Cohen SB, Lane NE, Palmer W, Shergy W, Zhou L, et al. Effects of denosumab on bone mineral density and bone turnover in patients with rheumatoid arthritis receiving concurrent glucocorticoids or bisphosphonates. Ann Rheum Dis. 2010 May;69(5):872–5.
91. Mok CC, Ho LY, Ma KM. Switching of oral bisphosphonates to denosumab in chronic glucocorticoid users: A 12-month randomized controlled trial. Bone. 2015 Jun;75:222–8.
92. Gladman DD, Dhillon N, Su J, Urowitz MB. Osteonecrosis in SLE: Prevalence, patterns, outcomes and predictors. Lupus. 2018 Jan;27(1):76–81.
93. Gladman DD, Urowitz MB, Chaudhry-Ahluwalia V, Hallet DC, Cook RJ. Predictive factors for symptomatic osteonecrosis in patients with systemic lupus erythematosus. J Rheumatol. 2001 Apr;28(4):761–5.
94. Calvo-Alén J, McGwin G, Toloza S, Fernández M, Roseman JM, Bastian HM, et al. Systemic lupus erythematosus in a multiethnic US cohort (LUMINA): XXIV. Cytotoxic treatment is an additional risk factor for the development of symptomatic osteonecrosis in lupus patients: Results of a nested matched case-control study. Ann Rheum Dis. 2006 Jun;65(6):785–90.
95. Zhang K, Zheng Y, Jia J, Ding J, Wu Z. Systemic lupus erythematosus patients with high disease activity are associated with accelerated incidence of osteonecrosis: A systematic review and meta-analysis. Clin Rheumatol. 2018 Jan;37(1):5–11.
96. Davidson JE, Fu Q, Rao S, Magder LS, Petri M. Quantifying the burden of steroid-related damage in SLE in the Hopkins Lupus Cohort. Lupus Sci Med. 2018;5(1):e000237.
97. Hussein S, Suitner M, Béland-Bonenfant S, Baril-Dionne A, Vandermeer B, Santesso N, et al. Monitoring of osteonecrosis in systemic lupus erythematosus: A systematic review and meta-analysis. J Rheumatol. 2018 Oct 45(10):1462–76.
98. Alarcón GS, Calvo-Alén J, McGwin G, Uribe AG, Toloza SM, Roseman JM, et al. Systemic lupus erythematosus in a multiethnic cohort: LUMINA XXXV. Predictive factors of high disease activity over time. Ann Rheum Dis. 2006 Sep;65(9):1168–74.
99. Kent T, Davidson A, Newman D, Buck G, D'Cruz D. Burden of illness in systemic lupus erythematosus: Results from a UK patient and carer online survey. Lupus. 2017 Sep;26(10):1095–100.

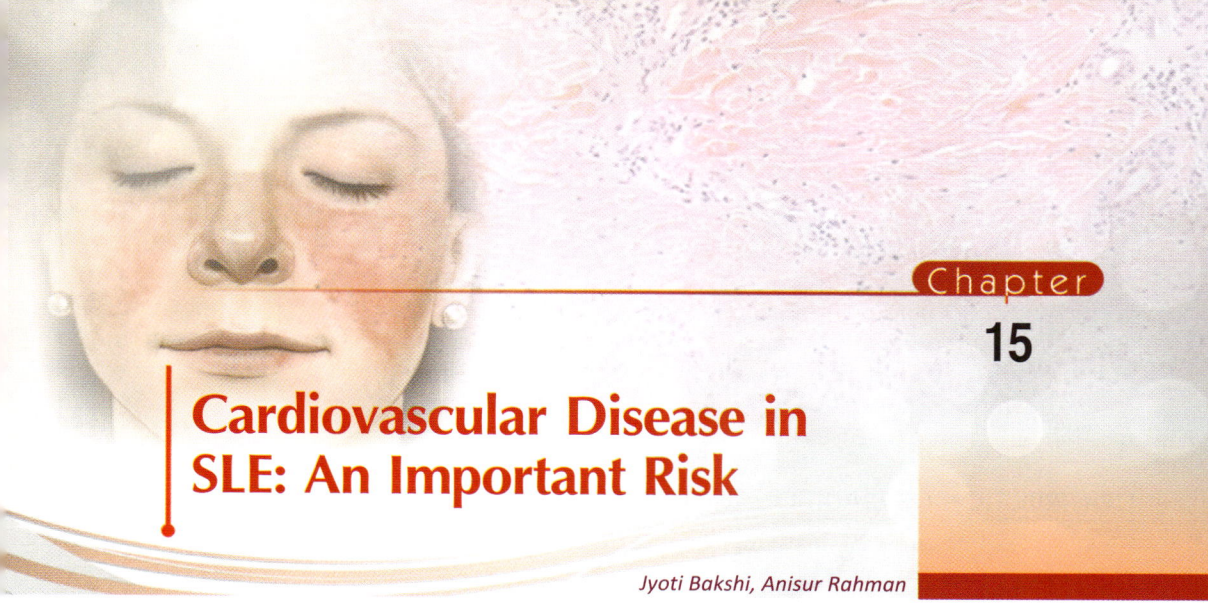

Cardiovascular Disease in SLE: An Important Risk

Jyoti Bakshi, Anisur Rahman

INTRODUCTION

Imagine you are in a pop concert, and the arena is filled with thousands of young women. How many of these young women will develop CVD within the next 10 years? The answer should be a very small number. Now imagine all these young women have SLE, and the answer is different. A surprising number of women with SLE develop CVD compared to healthy people of the same age and gender. A 5–10 fold increased risk of developing CVD in SLE patients has been reported in comparison to age–sex matched controls from epidemiological data from all over the world.[1] A particularly striking fact is that the presence of SLE in women between the ages of 35–44 increases the risk by 50 times.[2] However, knowing which patients with SLE will develop CVD and how best to manage these patients remains a pertinent and challenging question. In this chapter we aim to draw attention to the epidemiology, possible mechanisms, potential management strategies and evolving research concerning management of CVD risk in patients with SLE.

INCREASED PREVALENCE OF ATHEROSCLEROSIS AND CVD

A large multinational study of 9547 patients with SLE reported a quarter (313 out of 1255) deaths being caused by CVD.[3] The greatest relative risk for SLE patients is premenopausal. In the subpopulation of patients with SLE, who develop CVD, the average age of the first event is only 49 years;[4] which is much younger than in the general population, where the first CVD event typically occurs over the age of 60.

As well as established events, it has also been shown in a number of different studies using a variety of imaging techniques (such as vascular ultrasound and electron beam tomography) that lupus patients also have a considerably increased prevalence of asymptomatic atherosclerotic plaque compared to healthy controls. Studies from multiple centres in different countries have shown that 30–40% of patients with SLE have carotid plaque detectable by ultrasound.[5,6] Carotid ultrasound (US) may be an effective non-invasive method of detecting subclinical disease. Manzi and colleagues have shown that carotid measures on US can be used to predict the development of CVD in SLE patients. In 392 women with SLE followed for a mean of 8 years they showed that higher intimal-medial thickness (IMT) or presence of plaque at baseline predicted development of CHD or stroke over the next 10 years in multivariable analysis.[7] Most of these studies have been done in European and North American populations. The population studied by Manzi, et al. were predominantly a white (87%) population. Very little is known about Asian Indian SLE patients and CVD, despite Indians having a high prevalence of the metabolic syndrome and developing early atherosclerosis.[8] A study by Bhatt SP, et al. showed that Asian Indian SLE patients had significantly thicker carotid artery IMT and more plaque than healthy controls. The SLE patients were young with relatively short disease duration (age 31.6±10.05, median 30.5 years; disease duration 52.3±36.7, median 46 months).[9]

CONTRIBUTION OF TRADITIONAL CVD RISK FACTORS IN PATIENTS WITH SLE

CVD is a leading cause of death in Indian women and in both men and women CVD develops at an earlier age compared to Western populations.[10] Studies have shown that at younger ages, traditional CVD risk factors such as abdominal obesity, hypertension and diabetes are higher among Indians compared to other ethnic groups.[11] Smoking rates are lower in Indian women (less than 3%) compared to the west (10–19%), but they are growing at a faster rate than among Indian men.[12]

Conventional risk factors that contribute to CVD in the general population are common in SLE. Hypercholesterolemia is found in 34–51% of patients with SLE.[13] The "lupus pattern" of dyslipidemias is characterized by elevated levels of very low density lipoprotein (VLDL) and triglycerides and low high-density lipoprotein (HDL) levels.[14] Raised total cholesterol is predictive of future CHD in SLE.[15] SLE patients are more likely to be hypertensive than the general population due to steroid therapy use and the presence of renal impairment.[13] Most studies show that at least 10% of SLE patients continue to smoke.[6] 5 to 7% of patients with SLE develop diabetes and patients with SLE are more likely to develop diabetes than the general population.[13]

Whilst these traditional CVD risk factors may well account for some of the increased risk of developing CVD in patients with SLE, they fail to fully explain all of this risk. Studies have shown that traditional CVD risk calculators based on the Framingham equations grossly underestimate CVD risk in patients with lupus.[15,16] In a study of 263 Canadian patients with SLE, of whom 50 suffered CVD events over a mean 8.6 year period of follow-up, Esdaile, et al. reported a 7–10 fold increased risk of CVD even after adjusting for Framingham risk factors.[17]

This does not mean that the traditional risk factors can be ignored. In a large multi-center study of the Systemic Lupus International Collaborative Clinics (SLICC) inception cohort, Urowitz, et al. found that among 1249 patients followed for a mean of 8 years there were 31 atherosclerotic events. In univariate analysis all the factors significantly associated with increased risk of atherosclerosis were generic, rather than SLE-specific. These included male gender, increased age, smoking, hypertension and family history of CVD but in multivariable analysis only non-modifiable risk factors—age and male gender—remained significant.[18]

The QRISK3 score has been recently published and validated as a cardiovascular disease risk algorithm for use in the general population. Nearly 364,000 incident cases of cardiovascular disease were identified in the derivation cohort during follow-up arising from 50.8 million person years of observation. QRISK3 includes SLE as one of the factors used to calculate risk so using it would, by definition, increase the calculated risk scores in patients with SLE,[19] perhaps making it easier to recommend treatment. The QRISK3 model has limitations like exclusion of patients who were on statins at baseline, thus potentially excluding a group of patients that may be at higher risk. Additionally, within a cohort of patients with SLE, the added score attributed to SLE is a constant factor for all patients, so that QRISK3 alone may not be helpful in distinguishing that subgroup of SLE patients who are at the highest risk of developing CVD.

In conclusion, we know that conventional CVD risk factors play some role in the development of CVD in patients with SLE and it is important to advise patients not to smoke and optimize management of hypertension and hyperlipidaemia. However, many patients with SLE who develop CVD do not have these risk factors and would not have high predicted risk of CVD even using QRISK3. Therefore, it is also important to study the influence of disease-related immunological factors.

SLE DISEASE-RELATED FACTORS INCLUDING EFFECT OF DRUGS

In one study, a six-point elevation in the SLE–disease activity index (SLEDAI) score over 1 year was associated with a 5% increase in CVD risk over 2 years, suggesting that the presence of active inflammatory disease mitigates a higher CVD risk.[20] Renal disease is common in SLE patients. Renal disease is independently associated with an increased CVD risk and also contributes through the increased risk of hypertension and diabetes. Nearly 50% of deaths in patients with renal lupus are attributed to CVD.[21]

The contribution of corticosteroids to an increased CVD risk is well-known from their adverse metabolic effects such as hypertension, diabetes, dyslipidemia and obesity. Ever-use of steroids and longer duration of use have been associated with an increased risk of CVD.[2] Patients with higher cumulative doses of steroids are also highly likely to be a subset with a higher inflammatory burden. Whether corticosteroids increase risk of atherosclerosis directly or causally through the increased risk of traditional CVD risk factors remains to be determined.[22]

Hydroxychloroquine has been shown to have cardioprotective benefits in SLE. Studies have shown lipid lowering effects (total cholesterol, low-density lipoprotein and triglycerides)[23] and lower mean glucose levels.[24] The protective effect of HCQ on the vasculature may be partly related to its ability to inhibit aPL-mediated platelet activity. SLE patients on HCQ have been found to have less carotid plaque than those not on HCQ.[6]

IMMUNOLOGICAL FACTORS

Central to the pathogenesis of atherosclerosis are inflammation and lipid dysfunction. These mechanisms are also dysregulated in lupus and immune factors have been postulated to contribute to this dysregulation. Inflammation plays a role in both atherosclerotic plaque formation and plaque rupture that occurs during an acute event.[25]

SLE is characterized by lipid defects and chronic inflammation. The idea of lipids being central to atherosclerosis and SLE patients harbouring dyslipidemias has directed a focus towards abnormal lipids in SLE as a possible pathway for CVD. SLE patients have been found to have dysfunctional pro-inflammatory HDL cholesterol which may accelerate low-density lipoprotein oxidation and atherosclerosis.[26] Another component of lipids, apo-lipoprotein 1 (ApoA1), the main constituent of HDL has also been a focus of investigation. Anti-apoA1 antibodies could interfere with the protective functions of HDL and could thus promote development of CVD. Raised anti-apoA1 levels have been associated with both current and persistent disease activity in both prospective and retrospective analyses and in longitudinal and cross-sectional studies in SLE.[27] Elevated levels of anti-apoA1 antibodies have been associated with acute coronary syndromes in the general population and patients with rheumatoid arthritis.[28] No link between anti-apoA1 levels and CVD in patients with SLE has yet been established.

Invariant natural killer T-cells (*i*NKT) are another immunological factor that links SLE and lipids. Uniquely, they respond to lipid antigens presented by the CD1d molecule on antigen presenting cells[29] and are specialised immune cells that make up less than 0.1% of peripheral blood mononuclear cells. These cells may play a role in both autoimmunity and atherosclerosis.

Studies have shown that *i*NKTcells are reduced in number and have impaired function in SLE suggesting a protective role in autoimmunity.[30] A pro-atherogenic role of *i*NKT cells has been shown in mouse models. Human studies however have suggested that *i*NKT cells may be protective in the early stages of atherosclerosis and promoting resolution.[31]

The role of *i*NKT cells in the development of subclinical atherosclerosis was studied in 100 patients with SLE without any history of prior CVD using vascular ultrasound.[31] In keeping with previous studies, 36% of patients in this cohort had subclinical plaque.[6] SLE patients with pre-clinical plaque had an anti-inflammatory profile characterized by increased activation and IL-4 production. This correlated with serum lipid expression levels. Serum from patients with sub-clinical plaques activated *i*NKT cells to induce a M2 (anti-inflammatory macrophage polarization) phenotype *in vitro*. This was not seen in patients with SLE who had a history of CVD. In this group, they had a low frequency of *i*NKT cells with, increased CD8+, reduced CD69 expression and low expression of IL-4 and IFN-γ. SLE patients with a history of CVD also had an increased number of pro-inflammatory monocytes (CD14++CD16+). These findings suggest that during the early phase of atherosclerosis, serum lipids drive *i*NKT cells towards anathero-protective role.

Identification of immunological factors may in the future enable us to identify the sub-group of lupus patients who are at a higher risk of CVD to enable risk stratification and more stringent control of disease activity and traditional CVD risk factors (Fig. 15.1).

MANAGEMENT OF CVD RISK IN PATIENTS WITH SLE—NOW AND IN THE FUTURE

Let us return to our imaginary crowd of young women with SLE at a pop concert. How can we save as many of them as possible from developing premature CVD? First of all, we should make a detailed assessment of their traditional risk factors and manage them appropriately. SLE subjects should be screened annually for cardiac risk factors—a Boston cohort showed that only 26% of patients had 4 cardiac risk factors assessed annually.[26]

Although there are currently no formal published guidelines as to how to manage traditional CVD risk factors in patients with SLE, we would advocate a target-based approach. As SLE is a very high risk condition for CVD it can be viewed as a "coronary heart disease equivalent" and therefore we propose that targets used for conditions such as diabetes should also be used in SLE[13] (Table 15.1).

At present, carotid US is not easily available and the results are operator-dependent so that it cannot be used routinely in the management of CVD risk in patients with SLE. However, in future, we envisage the possibility that a combination of immunological factors (e.g. *i*NKT function, pro-inflammatory HDL, anti-apoA1 antibodies) and QRISK3 scores

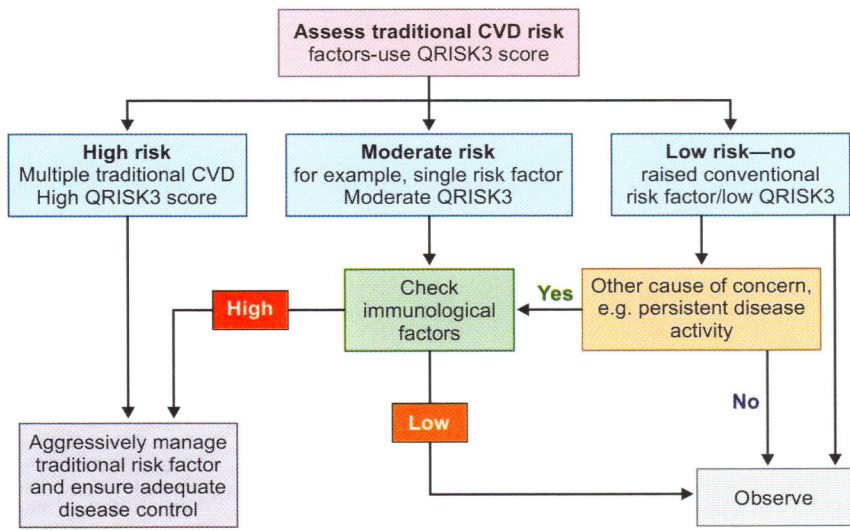

Fig. 15.1: Future algorithm for identifying patients at high risk at every clinic visit. If resources are available, carotid US could be used as an adjunct with immunological factors for the moderate risk group

	Table 15.1: Assessment of traditional CVD risk factors in SLE[13]	
Risk factor	*Frequency of assessment*	*Target and treatment*
Smoking	Annual	Counselling to stop, referral to cessation clinics. Drug treatments, e.g. nicotine replacement therapy.
Cholesterol	Annual fasting lipids namely total, HDL, LDL, and triglycerides	LDL cholesterol key lipid parameter; 1. LDL cholesterol <2.6 mmol/L no action review annually 2. LDL 2.6–3.4 mmol/L therapeutic lifestyle changes—diet and weight reduction 3. LDL >3.4 mmol/L or if still >2.6 despite lifestyle modification—drug therapy, e.g. statin
Body mass index	Annual	>25 kg/m² (over weight)—if related to steroid then adjust steroid dose, lifestyle modifications, exercise programmes, dietary education, reducing alcohol. If above fail then consider drug treatment
Diabetes mellitus	Each visit as part of SLE assessment—urine sample Random glucose—annually at least Monitor those on high-dose steroids more closely	DM diagnosed in presence of fasting glucose ≥7 mmol/L or random blood glucose or ≥11 mmol/L

could be used to improve accurate identification of SLE patients who would benefit from carotid US or whose CVD risk factor should be managed aggressively even without imaging. This idea is summarized in Fig. 15.1.

CONCLUSION

The increased risk of CVD in SLE has been well established. The contribution of traditional CVD risk factors and SLE-disease control are important facets in the management of CVD. Future work should focus on immunological biomarkers that may help alongside using traditional approaches and imaging to risk stratify these patients for early aggressive intervention and may even lead to the development of targeted therapies.

REFERENCES

1. Bruce IN. 'Not only...but also': factors that contribute to accelerated atherosclerosis and premature coronary heart disease in systemic lupus erythematosus. Rheumatol Oxf Engl. 2005 Dec;44(12):1492–502.
2. Manzi S, Meilahn EN, Rairie JE, Conte CG, Medsger TA, Jansen-McWilliams L, et al. Age-specific incidence rates of myocardial infarction and angina in women with systemic lupus erythematosus: comparison with the Framingham Study. Am J Epidemiol. 1997 Mar 1;145(5):408–15.
3. Bernatsky S, Boivin J-F, Joseph L, Manzi S, Ginzler E, Gladman DD, et al. Mortality in systemic lupus erythematosus. Arthritis Rheum. 2006 Aug;54(8):2550–7.
4. Elliott JR, Manzi S, Edmundowicz D. The role of preventive cardiology in systemic lupus erythematosus. Curr Rheumatol Rep. 2007 May;9(2):125–30.
5. Manzi S, Selzer F, Sutton-Tyrrell K, Fitzgerald SG, Rairie JE, Tracy RP, et al. Prevalence and risk factors of carotid plaque in women with systemic lupus erythematosus. Arthritis Rheum. 1999 Jan;42(1):51–60.
6. Roman MJ, Shanker B-A, Davis A, Lockshin MD, Sammaritano L, Simantov R, et al. Prevalence and correlates of accelerated atherosclerosis in systemic lupus erythematosus. N Engl J Med. 2003 Dec 18;349(25):2399–406.
7. Thompson T, Sutton-Tyrrell K, Wildman RP, Kao A, Fitzgerald SG, Shook B, et al. Progression of carotid intima-media thickness and plaque in women with systemic lupus erythematosus. Arthritis Rheum. 2008 Mar;58(3):835–42.
8. Misra A, Vikram NK. Insulin resistance syndrome (metabolic syndrome) and obesity in Asian Indians: evidence and implications. Nutr Burbank Los Angel Cty Calif. 2004 May;20(5):482–91.
9. Bhatt SP, Handa R, Gulati GS, Sharma S, Pandey RM, Aggarwal P, et al. Atherosclerosis in Asian Indians with systemic lupus erythematosus. Scand J Rheumatol. 2006 Apr;35(2):128–32.
10. Chow CK, Patel AA. Women's cardiovascular health in India. Heart. 2012 Mar 15;98(6):456–9.
11. Huffman MD, Prabhakaran D, Osmond C, Fall CHD, Tandon N, Lakshmy R, et al. Incidence of cardiovascular risk factors in an Indian urban cohort results from the New Delhi birth cohort. J Am Coll Cardiol. 2011 Apr 26;57(17):1765–74.
12. Goel S, Tripathy JP, Singh RJ, Lal P. Smoking trends among women in India: Analysis of nationally representative surveys (1993–2009). South Asian J Cancer. 2014 Oct;3(4):200–2.
13. Wajed J, Ahmad Y, Durrington PN, Bruce IN. Prevention of cardiovascular disease in systemic lupus erythematosus—proposed guidelines for risk factor management. Rheumatol Oxf Engl. 2004 Jan;43(1):7–12.
14. Borba EF, Bonfá E. Dyslipoproteinemias in systemic lupus erythematosus: Influence of disease, activity, and anticardiolipin antibodies. Lupus. 1997;6(6):533–9.
15. Rahman P, Urowitz MB, Gladman DD, Bruce IN, Genest J. Contribution of traditional risk factors to coronary artery disease in patients with systemic lupus erythematosus. J Rheumatol. 1999 Nov;26(11):2363–8.

16. Bessant R, Hingorani A, Patel L, MacGregor A, Isenberg DA, Rahman A. Risk of coronary heart disease and stroke in a large British cohort of patients with systemic lupus erythematosus. Rheumatol Oxf Engl. 2004 Jul;43(7):924–9.

17. Esdaile JM, Abrahamowicz M, Grodzicky T, Li Y, Panaritis C, du Berger R, et al. Traditional Framingham risk factors fail to fully account for accelerated atherosclerosis in systemic lupus erythematosus. Arthritis Rheum. 2001 Oct;44(10):2331–7.

18. Urowitz MB, Gladman D, Ibañez D, Bae SC, Sanchez-Guerrero J, Gordon C, et al. Atherosclerotic vascular events in a multinational inception cohort of systemic lupus erythematosus. Arthritis Care Res. 2010 Jun;62(6):881–7.

19. Hippisley-Cox J, Coupland C, Brindle P. Development and validation of QRISK3 risk prediction algorithms to estimate future risk of cardiovascular disease: Prospective cohort study. BMJ. 2017 May 23;357:j2099.

20. Karp I, Abrahamowicz M, Fortin PR, Pilote L, Neville C, Pineau CA, et al. Recent corticosteroid use and recent disease activity: Independent determinants of coronary heart disease risk factors in systemic lupus erythematosus? Arthritis Rheum. 2008 Feb 15;59(2):169–75.

21. Appel GB, Pirani CL, D'Agati V. Renal vascular complications of systemic lupus erythematosus. J Am Soc Nephrol JASN. 1994 Feb;4(8):1499–515.

22. Elliott JR, Manzi S. Cardiovascular risk assessment and treatment in systemic lupus erythematosus. Best Pract Res Clin Rheumatol. 2009 Aug;23(4):481–94.

23. Wallace DJ, Metzger AL, Stecher VJ, Turnbull BA, Kern PA. Cholesterol-lowering effect of hydroxychloroquine in patients with rheumatic disease: Reversal of deleterious effects of steroids on lipids. Am J Med. 1990 Sep;89(3):322–6.

24. Petri M. Hydroxychloroquine use in the Baltimore Lupus Cohort: Effects on lipids, glucose and thrombosis. Lupus. 1996 Jun;5 Suppl 1:S16-22.

25. Hansson GK. Inflammation, atherosclerosis, and coronary artery disease. N Engl J Med. 2005 Apr 21;352(16):1685–95.

26. McMahon M, Grossman J, Skaggs B, Fitzgerald J, Sahakian L, Ragavendra N, et al. Dysfunctional proinflammatory high-density lipoproteins confer increased risk of atherosclerosis in women with systemic lupus erythematosus. Arthritis Rheum. 2009 Aug;60(8):2428–37.

27. O'Neill SG, Giles I, Lambrianides A, Manson J, D'Cruz D, Schrieber L, et al. Antibodies to apolipoprotein A-I, high-density lipoprotein, and C-reactive protein are associated with disease activity in patients with systemic lupus erythematosus. Arthritis Rheum. 2010 Mar;62(3):845–54.

28. Vuilleumier N, Reber G, James R, Burger D, de Moerloose P, Dayer J-M, et al. Presence of autoantibodies to apolipoprotein A-1 in patients with acute coronary syndrome further links autoimmunity to cardiovascular disease. J Autoimmun. 2004 Dec;23(4):353–60.

29. Cho Y-N, Kee S-J, Lee S-J, Seo S-R, Kim T-J, Lee S-S, et al. Numerical and functional deficiencies of natural killer T cells in systemic lupus erythematosus: Their deficiency related to disease activity. Rheumatol Oxf Engl. 2011 Jun;50(6):1054–63.

30. van Puijvelde GH, van Wanrooij EJ, Hauer AD, de Vos P, van Berkel TJ, Kuiper J. Effect of natural killer T cell activation on the initiation of atherosclerosis. Thromb Haemost. 2009 Aug;102(2):223–30.

31. Smith E, Croca S, Waddington KE, Sofat R, Griffin M, Nicolaides A, et al. Cross-talk between iNKT cells and monocytes triggers an atheroprotective immune response in SLE patients with asymptomatic plaque. Sci Immunol. 2016 Dec 2;1(6).

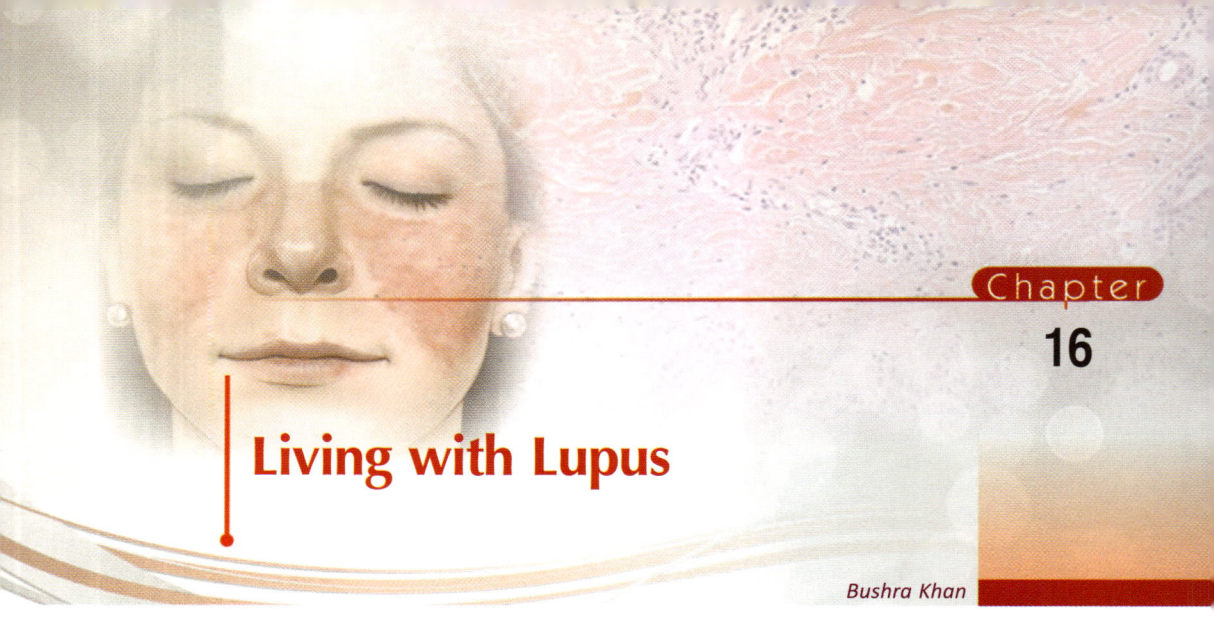

Living with Lupus

Bushra Khan

I was first diagnosed with lupus when I was in the 8th grade, at the ripe old age of 13, and I can honestly say that the process of actually getting a diagnosis from a doctor was harder on me emotionally than the diagnosis itself. I've had joint problems, fever, fainting spells, and general issues with falling ill for almost a year. I'd even developed the classic butterfly rash that comes along with lupus. I was given typhoid medication in the initial months because doctors were always convinced I have typhoid or flu. But, then my condition had deteriorated and I was referred to AIIMS or SGPGI. Being from small town was one of the reasons why doctors in my town did not know of lupus in 90s. After, I was hospitalised in SGPGI, it took a month or so of laboratory tests to confirm the diagnosis—SLE nephritis.

I was an extremely active, social and 'normal' pre-teen. I went from playing outdoor game, to not being able to walk. As a teenager, I remember distinctly feeling like my lupus was a burden to my family. It made me incredibly sad and my self-worth hit an all-time low. Feelings of sadness, worry, worthlessness, anxiety and hopelessness are normal feelings to have in the beginning. However, those feelings had become all-consuming and I couldn't eat (or overeat) and used to sleep all day. My circle of friends went on living their lives and I was catapulted into the hospital world. Instead of school teachers, I had doctors and specialists. Instead of social events, I had hospitalisations and clinic visits. Instead of cool clothes, I had hospital gowns and IVs. It rocked my world.

When you hear what lupus can do, and what it has done to people, it changes your perspective. Then, in a blink of an eye, you have lupus. You see what lupus has done to not only your body, but also your life, and as soon as you are diagnosed with this disease, you blame it. You feel that you have no control. Or at least that's how I felt in the beginning of my lupus story. Some days—on the bad days—I still feel that way. But when you have lupus—the disease that isn't curable, that can attack anywhere at any time, a disease that gives you a lot of bad days and good days—it makes your good days so precious, and you thank God for those days. It makes you stop and take life day-by-day; it makes you slow down; and, in my case, it makes me sleep all-day.

Circa after 4 years of lupus treatment, my lupus was in remission and I stopped taking prescribed medication on my own. However, continued the regular follow-ups with rheumatologist just to ensure my lupus hasn't flared up. I was off medication for almost 10 years, after which I had a relapse in the year 2014. This time lupus had affected my digestive system along with kidney, which wasn't that severe as I have always been observant of any change in my body physiologically. However, I was still not convinced to start oral medication. I was counselled on how important it is for me to take medication as prescribed since lupus could only be controlled and not cured. Also, by this time I had gained weight because of water retention owing to kidney problem. This whole episode had taken a toll not just on my heath but also on my job. But I learnt the hard way that how important it is for us to take medicines to keep lupus in control.

So, this time I decided to make lifestyle changes along with medication—I started working out and eating healthy food. I recommend everyone, especially with lupus, to have some sort of physical activity since this worked as a miracle in my life. Today I am free of joints pain, chest pain, and feel comparatively less fatigued.

The real challenge comes at my workplace—the stress and the struggle to educate people on what it is like to live with lupus. I have faced many people, including my family members, who doubt the veracity of my illness, believing it is all in my head. This is extremely painful and frustrating, causing anger and resentment. Thankfully I have a boss who understands what autoimmune diseases are like and what they can do to someone—I am provided with flexibility at work. This arrangement has helped me a lot in terms of managing my professional life with lupus.

However, because lupus is so very unpredictable, I have anxiety and fears about what is to come—how will it affect my body later? Will it get worse? Will I be able to take care of my needs both financially and physically in the coming years?

Still lupus has made me stronger. It has made me appreciate my good days and made me grow up and find myself. I am thankful for this lupus journey because it has brought so many people into my life that I would have never met otherwise—the most generous doctors. I try to raise awareness of this silent disease that not many understand. On the outside, most of us look happy and healthy, but on the inside we are fighting for our lives. I may have lupus, but lupus does not have me.

Index